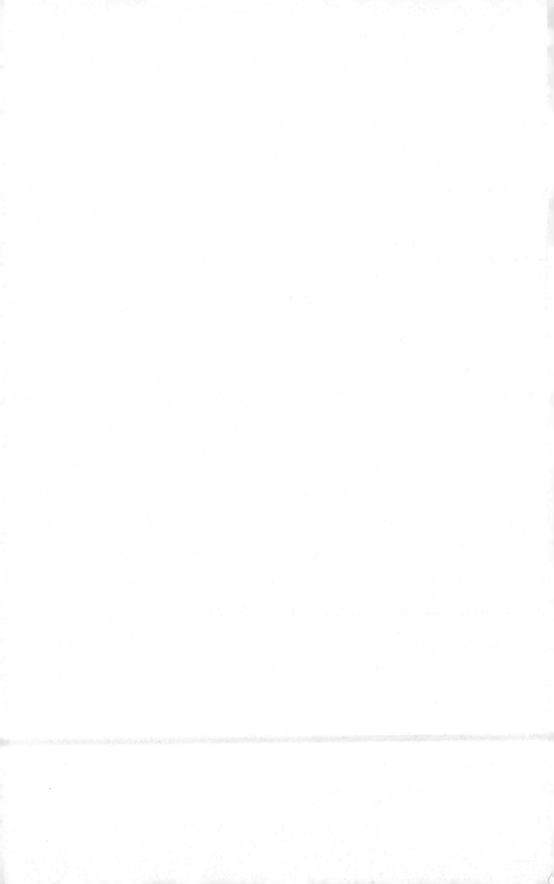

Praise for
Becoming Dead Right

"Parker gently leads us to examine the serious and un-discussed topic of death in this country by focusing on the lives of Gail, Crosby, Bea, and others who teach us that the end of our lives can be meaningful. This book is filled with poetry, stories, wisdom, and common sense that can help boomers, students, caregivers, and policy makers understand their own aging and realize that our society can—and should—make important changes that can ensure safe, dignified, individualized care at the end of our lives."
 —Alice H. Hedt, Executive Director
   National Citizens Coalition for Nursing Home Reform
   Washington, DC

"*Becoming Dead Right* gives us a blueprint for how we should approach dying and death. The author, through her impelling personal experiences as a hospice volunteer and her descriptive details of how each individual claims death, enfolds the reader into the many short stories that make us understand what hospice is all about."
 —Karyne Jones, President and CEO
   National Caucus and Center on Black Aged, Inc.
   Washington, DC

"Before I read this book, I knew very little about hospice care. Reading this book was extremely enlightening. It is so interesting and well written that I could hardly put it down. While maintaining universal appeal, perspectives of people of color are emphasized. I highly recommend this book as a "must read" for every individual who has ever experienced the illness and death of a loved one or who ever will. That includes everyone."
 —Naomi Long Madgett, Ph.D.
   Poet Laureate of the City of Detroit, Michigan

"There is no better description of cross-generational bonding and mutual learning than is found in *Becoming Dead Right*. Parker opens an amazing door of possibility with her lucid description of the loving intersects between students and nursing home residents. Drawing deeply from her own vivid experiences with elders in her family, Ms. Parker makes the case for more formal attachments between schools and nursing homes, using the emergent pedagogy of service learning."

—James C. Kielsmeier Ph.D., President
National Youth Leadership Council
Saint Paul, MN

"Ms. Parker leans on her years as educator and hospice volunteer to challenge us to look beyond stereotypes that pigeonhole our beliefs about what the elderly and the young can do when given the opportunity. For many, this door of opportunity is opened by service-learning, a teaching and learning method that engages young people in solving problems within their schools and communities, as part of their academic studies or other intentional learning activities. Ms. Parker's book is a blueprint for action and an example of compassion that I hope many will read and also follow."

—Nelda Brown, Executive Director
National Service-Learning Partnership
  at the Academy for Educational Development
Washington, DC

"The author, an inner-city hospice volunteer, pits her humanity against the neglect, shame, guilt, and fear that death and terminal illness provoke in modern urbanites. She weaves the invaluable lessons that she had gleaned from her vast experience with loving but unflinching sketches of her charges, her own poetry, and scathing, compelling dialogs. It is an incredible read, suffused with the surrealism that is an inevitable part of daily life in slums and housing projects, hospitals and care centers."

—Sam Vaknin, PhD, author *Malignant Self-Love*

Becoming Dead Right

A Hospice Volunteer in Urban Nursing Homes

FRANCES SHANI PARKER

First Edition: September 2007

Library of Congress Cataloging-in-Publication Data

Parker, Frances Shani, 1945-
  Becoming dead right : a hospice volunteer in urban nursing homes / Frances Shani Parker. -- 1st ed.
        p. cm.
  Includes bibliographical references and index.
  ISBN-13: 978-1-932690-35-4 (pbk. : alk. paper)
  ISBN-10: 1-932690-35-2 (pbk. : alk. paper)
  1. Hospice care--Michigan--Detroit--Anecdotes. 2. Terminal care--Michigan--Detroit--Anecdotes. 3. Palliative treatment--Michigan--Detroit--Anecdotes. 4. Parker, Frances Shani, 1945- 5. Volunteer workers in terminal care--Michigan--Detroit--Anecdotes. I. Title.
  R726.8.P3556 2007
  362.17'5609774--dc22
                                2007011692

Distributed by:
Baker & Taylor, Ingram Book Group, New Leaf Distributing

Published by:
Loving Healing Press
5145 Pontiac Trail
Ann Arbor, MI 48105
USA

http://www.LovingHealing.com or
info@LovingHealing.com
Fax +1 734 663 6861

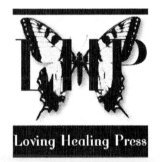

Loving Healing Press

Table of Contents

Poems

**To rainbow smiles for everyone
on both sides of Through**

Foreword

In his book, *Time of Our Lives: The Science of Human Aging*, Tom Kirkwood examines the biology of aging and notes that death is unfamiliar to so many young-adult and middle-aged individuals. Whereas in the 1880s only 74% of children born reached the age of 5, now over 99% do. Even at age 45, 96% of those born will survive to that age compared to barely over 50% in the 1880s. Thus, death is unfamiliar, uncomfortable, and increasingly a taboo topic. The dying are invisible to us, as they are mostly engaged in the dying process in hospitals or other institutions. Frances Shani Parker makes death and the dying a vivid part of life in her book *Becoming Dead Right: A Hospice Volunteer in Urban Nursing Homes.*

Ms. Parker describes the beginning of her journey into the world of hospice in the early chapters, engaging us in stories about men she knew who had HIV/AIDS and were dying. Her writing is excellent, and we see these men as whole individuals and not just as people dying. Ms. Parker brings her extraordinary gift of being able to see the many aspects of a person even when often these are covered up by pain, disease, or dementia. Section 1 of the book contains many stories of people and her experiences with them in nursing home settings. Ms. Parker astutely observes the challenges of nursing home staff as well and eloquently writes some of their stories. Ultimately, though, we are treated in this first section to Ms. Parker's love and compassion for those she serves and her humility in serving them. Her writing is tinged with profound respect for the individuals she worked with and helped. Each chapter closes with her lessons learned and her own poetry, much of which is compelling.

In part two, Ms. Parker broadens her book and gives advice and resources for the problems of caregiving, funerals, bereavement, hospice, and her dream for the future: Baby Boomer Haven. This part of the book is full of useful guides and facts, which will benefit all people caring for a loved one.

Ms. Parker was a school principal by profession. That title conjures up images of authority and power. It is thus striking that this book brings the stories of urban elders to the fore. Poverty, which so often makes people invisible, is not ignored here, but the stories of the human struggle, fear, kindnesses, and hopes predominate. This may be Ms. Parker's greatest gift to her readers: bringing to life people and events that are indeed so often invisible. This book is truly a gift. The writing is eloquent and powerful, and the stories are instructive and lasting. After finishing this book, I wanted to do more for other individuals who are dying, for as Ms. Parker so clearly imparts, the dying teach us so much about living well.

Peter A. Lichtenberg, Ph.D.
Director
Institute of Gerontology
Wayne State University
Detroit, Michigan

Introduction

The writing of this book rose from a restless literary hunger that confronted me with the urgency for promoting positive conversations about end-of-life healthcare, death, and nursing homes. An inner-city Detroit hospice volunteer for nine years, I ventured weekly into nursing home worlds where many patients lived final phases of their lives. Insights gained through my experiences became the food source for this book. Including both general and racial-ethnic minority perspectives, I wrote these stories, poems and commentaries to feed inspiration and information to readers about hospice, nursing homes, caregiving, health care disparities, death, and bereavement. Story themes and characters, some who are composites, are true. Dialogue approximates what was actually said. Names and descriptions are changed often for confidentiality.

Death is a necessary portion of life. Expressing our feelings, ideas, and plans regarding death and its challenges empowers us and enhances how well we adjust when faced with the mortality of others and ourselves. As America's buffet of populations continues to increase in age and diversity, important end-of-life concerns crave our attention. This book offers solutions for savoring, so we can all be nourished by gourmet satisfactions of dignified death journeys.

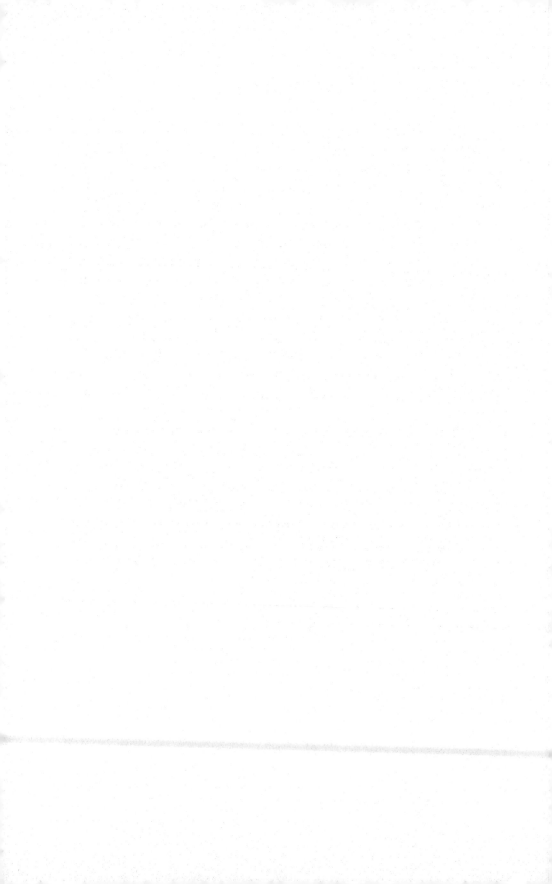

Part I:

Everybody's Story, Ready for the Telling

1 | Message from the Universe

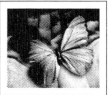

They watch me all the time, even when I use the bathroom," Jake lamented almost childlike. "They get mad when I don't leave the television on the cartoon channel. I can't sleep at night."

"Is that still going on? Are you still having those same problems? I thought things were getting better for you. What about your friend? Did you visit him to get your mind off this like we discussed a few weeks ago?" I asked.

"Yeah, I went to see him over the weekend, and they came, too," he responded wearily. "After I went inside, they made a big ruckus on the porch. It sounded like a whole bunch of them jumping, screaming, and laughing, just to get me all worked up. I kept running to the front door, opening it to catch them, but they would disappear too fast. My friend didn't understand what was going on. I tried my best to explain it to him. Finally, he told me I had to leave. I got the feeling he meant for good. What do I do now?"

Jake was a tall, brown, wiry man I knew from the neighborhood where I worked. He was well mannered and concerned about the community. Over a period of time, however, our infrequent conversations slowly began to revolve around his personal troubles. While I empathized with his sincere pleas for help, his stories became more bizarre each time we talked. We had discussed his unseen stalkers on several occasions. They chastised him about anything he said or did wrong, even small things like forgetting to hang up his washcloth after taking a shower, or leaving a light on when he left a room.

In the mornings, they stood outside his front door and hollered out what he was eating for breakfast. A mocking tone of laughter always accompanied their loud recitation of the breakfast menu. Jake waited for them to start hollering. Then he would jump up, run to the door, and swing

Knowing how stressed she was, I offered to write Jake's obituary for her. But Cherelyn felt that was something special she had to do herself. Writing in an informal voice, she soulfully described times she remembered with Jake. Sprinkled with exclamatory bursts of excitement like "Papa Jake's the greatest!" with a few typos and misspellings, it was the sweetest, from-the-heart obituary I've ever read. This young woman made of topnotch titanium was a living example of service being nothing but love in work clothes.

One quiet night, Jake lay quietly with a morphine pain patch on his chest. The damaged car of his life had reached its final destination. His previously fluctuating breathing eased slowly into a silent breeze. He closed his weary eyes for the last time as his engine stopped. The invisible demons left for good. His only stalker was Death.

Without either of us realizing it, Jake had introduced me to hospice care. I thought my experience with him was a once-in-a-lifetime occurrence. Like a flowing river, time passed while I labored to swim with the current. A year later, an acquaintance named Sam broke down crying in the parking lot after an exercise class we attended. I only knew him from the class, and he had stopped coming regularly. He told me he had been diagnosed with AIDS. He had kept this secret from others as long as he could. Because he had been absent so often from his job at a hardware store, he knew he couldn't go on working much longer. Family problems increased his need for help. His story resonated with déjà vu that I had no desire to revisit. Perplexed that a similar crisis could be happening to me again, I imagined familiar thorns invading my life's pruned rose garden.

Sam's stable mind concentrated on improving his health. He acknowledged he had AIDS and committed to fight for his life. He knew the time had come when he would have to tell others his secret. We both knew judgment and rejection would follow. I became a better listener by staying quiet while he rambled on about his plans for coping with his illness. He had already started his treatment regimen with a doctor. We went to his clinic appointments together sometimes. His nurse taught him a complex system of using pennies to keep track of the many medications he took around the clock.

Ongoing nausea and diarrhea suppressed most of his desire to socialize with others. He didn't seem to have many friends who were supporting him. Rotting teeth continued to add anguish to his growing list of illness issues. Hoping to get some help, he finally went to a dentist. The dentist examined his mouthful of decayed teeth and promptly announced, "Your teeth are all beyond saving. Any work done to replace them would be extensive and also expensive. There's no reason to go forward with this anyway. You have AIDS and probably won't be around much longer." Some words are better left unsaid or said differently, even when they might be true. The dentist's response angered Sam tremendously. He saw this as another hole in his rapidly sinking life raft.

Sam and his family disagreed on several matters. A few relatives had concerns about visiting him at his home. This bothered him because he felt they thought he would contaminate them with AIDS, even after he had explained to them that he wouldn't. In spite of these problems, there was definite support from a few family members who genuinely cared about him. On rare occasions, relatives came by to visit him. But usually he visited them at their homes.

Even though Sam mentioned seeing a few friends now and then, something was still missing. That something was communication with people who shared his condition, people who could hold on with him to the raft of one another, people who lived his inner turmoil like the rest of us didn't. He joined an AIDS support group and attended regular meetings that offered him opportunities to share his feelings with others who had AIDS.

Sam explained to me, "We go around the room, say our names, and talk about our problems. I thought my situation was bad, but I was surprised to hear about other peo-

with fellow Detroiters—mostly men, but also women and children—demonstrating commitment to a cause that would benefit humanity. Like many who participated, his involvement in the Million Man March ignited a fire in his spirit that reinforced his desire for creating positive changes in the future. It was a day of atonement and reconciliation, a day that called African American men to re-dedicate themselves to improving self, family, and community. Sam reached his goal that day and literally became one in a million.

Several weeks after Sam returned, he witnessed a large man brutally beating a woman in the street. He watched as long as he could and then resigned himself to get involved. Even though he was extremely weak, he persisted in trying to make the man stop by talking to him about the purpose of the Million Man March. Miraculously, the violence ended when the man freed the woman and listened. Sam told me later he was afraid of getting hurt, maybe even killed, but he still had to try to end the brutality. This was no small accomplishment for a thin man weighing about one hundred pounds. The march had empowered him to confront fear and take a stand for righteousness. I thought he had experienced his last joyous milestone.

One day, Sam told me that during the previous night, his head was spinning so fast, he didn't think it would stop until he reached outer space. That was the night he was sure he would die. When he tried to sit up, he fell back. Breathing seemed like lifting a boulder on his chest. Calling 911 or anyone else wasn't an option because his limp hand couldn't pick up the phone. He just lay there and waited for forever to pass. He felt so bad, he welcomed death. It was the closest he had ever come to giving up.

But daybreak came like it always did. Sunlight fingers of warmth crept through each gap in his bedroom blinds. Sleepy eyes opened slowly to a new awareness that he was still alive. Advancing bars of brightness gradually decorated his blanket. Sam smiled, knowing the falling sky was lifted for another day.

Death, sitting patiently outside Sam's bedroom door, still wasn't ready to leave with him. When his body was ravaged in the last stages of AIDS, Sam started taking new drugs called protease inhibitors that revolutionized the treatment of AIDS. The drug "cocktail" changed AIDS from being an automatic death sentence to a chronic, but manageable, disease. As a result of this major advance in medical science, the number of deaths due to AIDS began to decrease. The prevalence of AIDS continued to increase, however, because infected people were living longer, while new ones were continually being infected.

Thrilled with improvements in his life, Sam no longer needed to take various medications day and night. His skin cleared, leaving a physical glow that reflected his inner light. His weight increased, along with his strength. Looking almost as good as he had before the disease stole most of his physical assets, he spoke with new enthusiasm for life. The gnawing pain that had gripped his body daily like a gigantic fist became much easier to bear. Most of all, he felt reborn.

Physically and mentally, Sam rose from a grave of suffering after being closer to death than most people can ever imagine. He experienced the Lazarus Effect that normalized his blood cell count and restored him to productive living. I was elated to be an eyewitness to this wondrous resurrection. His life became a book with unread chapters of future possibilities, beginning with a network of new friends he had met through his support group. He and his friends helped one another, sharing a bond that only comes through experiencing mutual long-term tragedy.

Sam had come full circle through a medical maze of potential hopelessness. Although I felt optimistic about his future, I knew that the epidemic of HIV/AIDS in America continued to spread in all sectors of society, increasingly among women, young people, and people of color. Sam and I kept in touch until he stopped returning my phone calls. Intuitively, I knew he hadn't died. A few years later, we happened to see each other at a street festival. We spoke briefly, and he appeared to be doing well. When I asked him why he had stopped returning my phone calls, he responded, "I'm a busy man."

During the years before I saw Sam that day, my life had normalized. I thought about the two men whom I'd hardly known before I'd found out about their illnesses. Somehow I had woven my way through their forests of misery over a three-year period. Nobody was more surprised than I was. A person who never liked being around sick people had been transformed into an urban Florence Nightingale. What did it all mean? I listened to the universe for answers.

A few weeks later at a grocery store, I had a chance meeting with a friend named Ellen, whom I hadn't seen in quite awhile. She mentioned how much she enjoyed being a hospice volunteer, a form of volunteer work I hadn't seriously considered, even as I had been unknowingly performing it. Although I had been actively involved in various kinds of volunteer work most of my life, I felt her words inspire me, open my windows of curiosity higher. Later, it occurred to me that I had been a hospice volunteer for Jake and Sam. The following week, I saw a newspaper advertisement for hospice volunteer classes. I signed up for the training and felt my ship getting closer to harbor.

Remembering Jake

A lonely leper with AIDS,
you existed in a colony of inhumanity,
seldom felt life's caring caresses.
While demons dragged your body
through gutters of deterioration,
you relinquished your confused mind
to unseen terrorists who stalked,
robbed you of much needed rest.
I watched your painful decay,
witnessed abuses by family and friends
treating you like toxic waste.
Rare handfuls of love brought
limited smiles in your leper's life.
Sweet Death delivered your only peace.

—Frances Shani Parker

This poem was read at the 13th International AIDS Conference in South Africa. Jake was there in spirit, enjoying all the caring caresses he missed in life.

<table>
<tr><td>

2

</td><td>

Defining
Moment

</td><td>

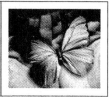

</td></tr>
</table>

I like educational settings where interesting ideas grab me by the collar, confront me with opportunities to learn and solve problems. But taking classes in volunteer hospice training seemed like an entirely different undertaking. Death was the ultimate topic. Most people don't even want to discuss death briefly. To take a whole course on people dying seemed strange. I was curious about how this subject would be taught. The class schedule included twenty hours of hospice training for certification. Some institutions require fewer hours.

My first class consisted of a dozen students from varied backgrounds. All were as eager as I was to learn what hospice entailed and what our future responsibilities might be. Looking around the room, I wondered what had motivated others to come. Had they been listening to the universe, too? Everyone had questions that needed answers. Our teacher reassured us that concerns would all be addressed as the class progressed. After a warm welcome and introductions, she introduced the history of the hospice movement. I learned how attitudes about aging and dying evolved through the years and led to a new approach to caring for the terminally ill.

Americans' tendency to strive for longevity, even when people are in the process of dying, is one reason the hospice movement in the United States has been slower to advance than in Europe. The hospice philosophy embraces support of the dying and their families through high-quality patient care physically, emotionally, socially, and spiritually. Because all of these areas are interwoven in patients' lives, they must be addressed as a unit during patients' treatments. Input from patients and primary caregivers involved in the plan of care is welcomed and respected. Hospice beliefs must be understood and accepted by all persons involved in hospice care, including patients, medical personnel, and caregivers.

Hospice care refers to non-aggressive treatment of patients who have been diagnosed as terminally ill. It is available for individuals who have a life expectancy considered to be in months, usually within six months. Cases are subject to renewal after the six-month period. Hospice neither hastens nor postpones death, a natural part of living. The primary focus of hospice care is to provide support and relief for patients. Palliative care, an approach for treating incurable illnesses, can be given no matter how long a patient is expected to live and while doctors are still seeking a cure. Relieving pain and other symptoms, palliative care extends the hospice philosophy to a larger population that can benefit earlier in the illness process. Ideally, it precedes hospice care.

I learned that hospice services should start as soon as the terminal phase of illness begins. Anyone can make a hospice referral, but doctors write the orders that begin official hospice care procedures. Patients or those legally in charge of making medical decisions for patients make the decision for beginning or ending hospice care. Depending on their health progress, patients can be discharged or re-admitted by the hospice team.

Patients with various kinds of illnesses, including AIDS, cancer, stroke, heart disease, dementia, and kidney disease are eligible for hospice care. Services are provided to patients whether they live in private homes, apartments, or group facilities. Medicare and most insurance plans pay for hospice care and cover people of all ages. Hospice pays for medications and provides supplies and equipment related to the hospice diagnosis.

Dying is a natural part of life, not something to be dreaded or feared. It is a process in which the body slows down and is a unique experience for each person. Several speakers joined the class periodically to share their expertise and answer questions. They gave interesting information about various aspects of hospice care such as the use of equipment in assisting patients. They described signs of dying such as decreased desire for food or fluids, increase or decrease in pain, or increased weakness in terminally ill patients.

The basic role of a hospice volunteer is to enhance the quality of life for patients during their end-of-life stages. Patients should be comfortable. Their bodies should serve as resting places for peace, so their deaths will be positive experiences. This allows them to know dignity during this critical time in their lives. Volunteers provide companionship and assistance with normal tasks such as letter writing and wheelchair rides. Another important service volunteers provide is advocacy for patients when they need it. For example, if a patient has not been fed or cleaned properly, a volunteer brings this to the attention of those who can correct the problem.

Fortunately, a volunteer does not work alone. A hospice team, consisting of a medical director, nurse, certified nurse aide (also called CNA or certified nursing assistant), social worker, dietitian, chaplain, and volunteer coordinator, is available to serve patients. Working together, members of the hospice team provide support in decisions regarding patients' total treatment during their last phase of life, including the implementation of patients' advanced directives. These are documents that give healthcare providers directions regarding patients' treatment preferences under certain circumstances. The hospice team provides not only medical support, but also social, nutritional, and spiritual support for patients and their families.

In order to work best with the team, I needed to know the various roles each team member played. These were explained as the class unfolded. The medical director manages clinical care. Volunteers work directly under a volunteer coordinator. She manages volunteers through recruitment, record keeping, training, assignments, and recognition of their contributions as volunteers. Nurses, with the assistance of nurse aides, work closely with the medical director and other doctors to facilitate patients' care. Dietitians address food-related concerns. Social workers help patients and their families with illness and death concerns. Chaplains assist with spiritual matters.

I listened to everything being said, wondering if my own philosophy matched those of the hospice program. At a personal level, I did not fear death. I assumed it would be a transition to a life better than this one. In that sense, I certainly didn't dread its coming. But a terminal illness has the potential for being a very difficult and painful journey for some people. Becoming a part of others' death journeys on a long-term basis presented another perspective. I had experienced this already with Jake and Sam. My ability to empathize with future patients would require frequent and intense use. Because I know I am a strong person, I felt certain I could succeed in my efforts to provide needed support. However, I still had a lot more to learn.

Class members were told to use the words "death" and "died," instead of euphemisms like "eternal rest" and "passed." As a child, I had noticed how people used indirect words when they spoke about death. Pets were "put to sleep" or "put down." Even jokingly, death was referred to as "kicking the bucket." These terms are still used today.

Society sends a strong message that dying is not a subject that should be embraced. Death is the elephant in the room that we pretend not to see until it sits heavily in our unfamiliar laps and pokes its intruding trunk in our faces. One certainty in life is that everyone will die. Many people refuse to say actual death words because of emotions the words generate. Others refuse to discuss death, particularly their own, even when they are well. Clouds of discomfort hover over death discussions. Fears center on how they will die, what happens after they die, and how their lives mattered. I knew I would have to analyze my own feelings thoroughly if I expected to help others.

During the class, I learned about various religious practices related to death. One of the beauties of diversity is having opportunities to become familiar with the cultural

Defining Moments

They come without warning,
grab us in chokeholds of change,
fling us into outer space
where past meets future.
In this realm resonating
with first-time knowledge,
we awaken wide-eyed,
infused with wisdom
to turn around, stand still,
or move forward with clarity.
No matter how they smack,
stroke, lift, drop, push, kiss,
or kick us to get our attention,
when they finish their mission,
we are permanently scarred.

—Frances Shani Parker

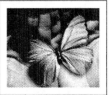
I had not been in a nursing home since my visits with Jake. Because he had AIDS and stayed in an isolated section, I had very little contact with the total nursing home environment there. Looking around my newly assigned nursing home, I noticed that most residents were African Americans, with smaller numbers of Caucasians and other racial and ethnic groups.

My first patient was a woman named Bea. In her nineties with serious heart trouble, she was usually confined to her bed or chair. Although she could walk briefly to her bathroom, there was a high likelihood that she would fall without assistance. Several times she did.

Bea couldn't participate in group activities, such as eating in the dining room, watching movies, or playing bingo games. In addition to her limited mobility, she also had trouble seeing, although she tried to recognize figures on the television. All of her relatives and friends lived out of town. Only a few visited occasionally. Hearing was also a problem, even with her hearing aid turned on. Struggling to chew solid food, she seldom wore her false teeth, which she didn't like. One of her favorite treats was a small bag of mini peanut butter sandwiches made with crackers.

Bea's mind seemed sharp as a switchblade. Interested in local and national news, she enjoyed expressing her spin on anything going on in the world. When she didn't understand something, she eagerly asked for an explanation. Unfortunately, she had no roommate who could join her in lively discussions. Lesley, her roommate, had deteriorated mentally with dementia. There was little communication between them. While Bea could call for help if something happened to Lesley, she worried about getting help for herself when she fell. Lesley's mind did not always perceive a crisis at hand and might ignore Bea's plight. Bea had few opportunities to really discuss all the topics in which she was interested. She looked forward to my weekly visits when I brought the outside world with me.

It didn't take long for me to figure out that how I interacted with Bea and other patients would depend a lot on intuition and good common sense. Although she could hardly hear the television or read normal-sized print, her mind still needed challenges. I knew she would appreciate exploring another world that would transcend her limitations in the nursing home. The wonderful world of books was the obvious answer. I contacted the Detroit Public Library and arranged for a bookmobile to bring her large-print books that would be her gateway to new adventures.

Every few weeks, Bea received a dozen books to read that were based on the interests she had indicated. Her favorite books were autobiographies, especially those about women, but she also enjoyed family stories that had good endings. Love stories were okay, as long as there was no sex or violence. Making a distasteful face, she stated, "I don't want to read any book that's got sex in it, and violence is just as bad. You don't need all that to tell a good story, even a love story. I don't know what the world is coming to with all this sex and violence."

Stories sometimes triggered memories about her childhood, later years, siblings, and friends. She kept her books stacked in a bag by her bed, so she could reach over and grab one whenever she wanted to read. Because the librarian had screened all the books to meet Bea's tastes, she hardly ever read one she didn't love. Each time I visited at the end of my school day, the first thing I did was listen to her oral book reviews, which she explained in great detail.

Once a patient named Michele, who also had dementia, strolled into Bea's room during the story telling. Like a human echo, she proceeded to repeat every sentence Bea said. At the same time, Lesley was having a lively two-way argument with an imaginary friend who was trying to force her to put on a sweater, so they could go outside and play.

"I like this story. It's about a boy and his family who live on a farm in Nebraska," explained Bea.

"I like this story. It's about a boy and his family who live on a farm in Nebraska," repeated Michele.

"You can't make me wear it if I don't want to. I bet I can. Put on this sweater right now," Lesley protested and demanded like two people arguing.

"The boy has a brown dog named Beacon that follows him everywhere he goes. This dog is very smart."

"The boy has a brown dog named Beacon that follows him everywhere he goes. This dog is very smart."

"You're not my boss. I told you I'm not going to put that sweater on. If you don't put it on, I won't play with you."

"One day the boy went fishing and forgot to bring his bait. He decided to find another way to get the fish to bite."

"One day the boy went fishing and forgot to bring his bait. He decided to find another way to get the fish to bite."

"I don't care if you don't play with me. I hate your guts! I hate your guts more than you hate mine!"

I sat listening to this gumbo of chatter from three different people sounding like four, each focused on her own compelling words. Somehow it was both interesting and amusing to observe this confusion. Bea asked me to make them stop interrupting her story, so I had to lead Michele out of the room. Lesley, of course, was sitting in her own bed, so she continued her dual discussion. Friends asked me how I could go to the nursing home after running an urban public school all day, and then put up with scenarios such as this. But it seemed like the most normal thing in the world, the nursing home world, that is.

Bea dictated letters for me to write to her few remaining friends and relatives. Most of them had died. She'd outlived two husbands and two of her children. She had stacks of stationery stored, along with stamps, in her drawers. These gifts from her family and friends encouraged her to correspond with them. She told them about her books, her family, and her hospice volunteer who wrote letters for her. When I went out of town, usually to educational conferences, I always sent Bea a postcard, so she would get some mail and see a colorful picture we could discuss later about my trip.

Because all students at my school participated in service learning, a teaching and learning approach that connects classroom learning with meeting community needs, groups of students went to visit Bea and other residents at the nursing home. Bea loved visits from children. She also craved information from me about television news that confused her. She said she had heard about the president of the United States doing something he had no business doing with a young woman. What was that all about? And why didn't Oprah and Stedman get married? Before I knew it, I had been her volunteer over two years.

But our visits weren't always pleasant. She told me about times she had fallen, and showed me bruises that decorated her arms like black and blue tattoos. Once I arrived to discover she hadn't eaten dinner because someone had forgotten to bring a dinner tray to her room. She didn't complain because, like many elderly people, she avoided "making trouble." Condiments like ketchup and mustard were often missing from her food tray, although she was allowed to eat them. I brought her a supply for her drawer.

Bea was concerned about herself and her family members. She worried about the dangers of falling, her increasing dependency on others, and whether her children were taking care of themselves. She fretted about the state of the world, how nothing was like it used to be, even the weather. A major concern was that she wouldn't be renewed as a hospice patient every time her case came up for evaluation. She appreciated the services and equipment she received through hospice. She had already lived way past her projected six-month life expectancy.

Because hospice team members were not always present at nursing home sites, hospice patients often received care from the nursing home staff. Unless these workers were trained well in hospice care procedures, they could sometimes give inappropriate service. Workers who were accustomed to focusing on restoring patients to good health had to make major readjustments helping patients die with dignity, while eliminating aggressive medical intervention. Staff shortages and high turnover impacted hospice care negatively. It was critical for staff members to understand that their active involvement in providing hospice support to patients was still needed, even to those who were dying or had advanced dementia. This was particularly important for staff who provided direct patient care on a regular basis.

I found staff morale low in many nursing homes where I worked, especially among nurse aides who provided front-line patient care helping patients with eating, dressing, toileting, and repositioning those who were immobile. I came to know some nurse aides well because we shared direct contact with patients. Most of them valued having a volunteer to help with patients. They also seemed to welcome the opportunity to express their concerns to someone who listened.

It was not unusual for a nurse aide to care for twelve or more patients, which is higher than their workload should be. On days with high absenteeism, the numbers of patients assigned to nurse aides increased. Unfortunately, the total amount of time allotted for aides to complete their tasks remained the same. They often worked under a great deal of pressure. Aides complained about low pay, difficult work conditions, being overworked, and not being appreciated.

A shortage in nurse aides had harmful consequences for some patients. This included being left in unchanged beds, not being fully clean, and not being assisted when help was required for eating. Some patients tried to feed themselves, using their hands when they couldn't see their eating utensils. Patients waiting for help sometimes stared at their food while it turned cold. Those with depression or dementia often had little interest in food. They needed someone to motivate them throughout the meal.

The shortage in nursing home employees reminded me of "troubled water" in the song "Bridge Over Troubled Water." Good combinations of family and friends often served as bridges over troubled water in nursing homes. Their ongoing visits to nursing homes led to more successful stays for residents there, particularly hospice patients surrounded by overworked employees.

"Hello, Sister, how are you today?" Lonnetta asked her eighty-year-old sister, who had been in the nursing home a few months. Although she appeared to be in a daze just before Lonnetta arrived, Sister recognized her immediately. Sister raised up her arms for a hug. I had seen her do this many times with others, including myself. She craved affection and actively sought it. Lonnetta squeezed the human pillow of Sister's chubby body.

"I'm fine. How are you today?" Sister giggled, happy to see her sister again.

"I'm always fine when I see you, Sister. My, don't you look cute in that red sweatsuit Aunt Gloria gave you for your birthday. Wish she could be here now. You know, you look just like her with those big bright eyes of yours. That's why she spoils you. She'll be so happy to spend time with you when she comes back in town."

Sister blushed, thinking about her doting aunt who always remembered her birthday. Aunt Gloria drove to Detroit from Atlanta to bring her gifts every year. Sister was basking in all the love she owned. She looked up sheepishly and asked, "Did you bring me something?"

"Did I bring you something? Now you know I always bring something special for my favorite and only sister. Today, I brought something that will make you grin like a jack-o-lantern. I brought two homemade cupcakes with chocolate icing. They even have happy faces I drew on them with pink icing. That's the way I like to see your face with a great big smile. What do you think of that?"

Sister's face lit up like she had won the lottery. She unwrapped her treats and hollered a huge, "Thank you!" Then she began eating each mouthful with enthusiasm, getting smears of dark brown sweetness around her honey-colored lips. Nothing could be better than Lonnetta's chocolate cupcakes! Her day was complete. Lonnetta had come to see her with the most fantastic food she could bring. This was the happiest day of her life. Tomorrow would be the happiest day of her life, too, when Lonnetta came to see her again. Making every day the happiest day of her life was Lonnetta's magic. Nobody made magic better than her sister.

Lonnetta's eyes surveyed Sister's condition. Was her hair combed? Were her clothes and linen clean? Did she appear overly medicated, hungry, depressed? Did she have any mysterious bruises? Lonnetta was evaluating Sister's care at the nursing home. Sister's mind was fading with dementia. It was hard for her to explain what went on when Lonnetta wasn't there. But if Lonnetta wasn't satisfied with her sister's care, she made her voice heard until the problem was corrected. She wasn't the kind of woman people wanted to agitate, particularly if she had already tried to work with them in a calm manner. With a black-belt tongue that could give air a whipping and make dinner trays tremble, Lonnetta didn't care what people thought when she finally caused a scene. All she cared about was Sister.

Employees at the nursing home knew that Lonnetta did an evaluation during her visits, which were scheduled at different times. They never could be sure about the time she would arrive. Conscious efforts were made by employees to be in compliance, even though they didn't always succeed. Lonnetta checked Sister's personal belongings located in her closet. Several caregivers had complained about patients' clothes being missing and a few gifts that had disappeared for unexplained reasons. One of my patient's portable oxygen tanks that had been provided by hospice turned up missing. I checked everywhere, but no one knew what happened to it. Another patient had an overcoat missing. He couldn't take a car trip with his family until he could borrow someone else's coat. Lonnetta took Sister's clothes home and washed them, just so she could keep track of them better.

Lonnetta was diligent about taking care of her sister, even though she was in a nursing home. Her method wasn't perfect, but it was better than no method at all. For the most part, it seemed to work, but there were still times when she had to raise the roof with a complaint about Sister's care. Sister was one of the lucky patients who had a persistent advocate with a personal interest in the quality of life to which she was entitled.

Because mobile patients roamed or wheeled themselves around the nursing homes, it was inevitable that I had contact with them. I met them when I walked in the halls, rode the elevator, or took my own patients on wheelchair rides. Halls were like narrow streets with tired wheelchairs sitting on the sidelines passing time, waiting for riders to decide on their next moves. Gradually, I became known as one of the regulars who visited from the outside world that patients had left behind. They had me shaking their hands, listening to make-believe adventures, and talking to their "baby" dolls.

"Hi, Susan, I see you're taking your baby with you to dinner," I said to a woman wearing a high wattage smile that her baldheaded "baby" inherited.

"Well, I want to take my baby out more. Everybody likes her, you know, especially me. She told me she was hungry."

"What's your baby's name?" I asked, exploring her reality.

She and the doll stared at each other, grinning as if they knew secrets from ancient times. And maybe they did. Susan looked at me, pointed to her baby and said, "She'll tell you her name when you come back with cookies."

I was a hospice volunteer who had found her niche in the first of many Detroit nursing homes—places where problems wrestle with solutions, hope struggles to keep the faith, and everybody has a special story ready for the telling.

Living Colors

A nursing home room
serves as your dining place.
Colors on a supper plate
charm century-old eyes.
Green, brown, white form
an aromatic rainbow
of bygone days that nourish,
thrill you with their stories.

When no one helps you eat,
you reach with forklike fingers.
Green tastes like memories
of grass tickling childhood toes.
Taste buds savor brownness
of a mahogany man who
hungered for your love.
Handfuls of August clouds
whisk you to a picnic,
hint at mashed potatoes.

A volunteer, I arrive to see
your smile smeared with dreams.
Each morsel of remembrance
has fed your starving mind.
Anchored in reality of meals
with special meanings,
your appetite is satisfied
with colors from the past.

—Frances Shani Parker

| 4 | # No Restful Stillness | 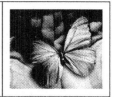 |

Dying a pain-free death is a basic principle of hospice care. I have known patients who died without excessive pain. When cure was no longer the focus, the dying process, with its naturally evolving stages, was facilitated in a manner that brought beauty to their personal letting go. Caregivers and others were in the presence of openness where they could listen with their hearts. The terminally ill often knew they were dying. They focused clearly on the outcome without the distractions of pain. Because they were given appropriate medical assistance, their bodies calmly ceased functioning. Death came in a gentle manner that brought perfect closure to life.

But successful hospice care depends greatly on the context in which it is provided. This includes people involved, pain management procedures, resources, and the general environment. I have also witnessed dying patients who were forced to fight toe-to-toe with terror. Some feared pain so much they welcomed death to end their misery. They stiffened, groaned, grimaced with looks of excruciating distress. Living became a series of tsunami pain waves that thrashed against their beach of peace. A tranquil death is not a privilege; it is an entitlement.

One of the worst cases I observed of someone dying in pain involved a man named Crosby who had AIDS. I had looked forward to becoming his volunteer. Because my first experiences performing hospice service had been with two men who had AIDS, I welcomed the opportunity to support another AIDS patient. Most of my patients had other illnesses.

But Crosby only stayed in hospice care a few days. The morning I met him, I heard his anguished moans before I entered his room. He appeared totally exhausted just dealing with suffering. Thunderbolts of lightning pain traveled throughout his feeble body. His eyes, shut in tight blind squints, told me there was no way we could carry on a conversation. I spoke calmly to him after alerting a staff member about his immediate misery. His groans softened, while his body rested in preparation for the next storm that would shower him with agony. I remember thinking that this was no way to die.

Looking around his sparse room, I noticed a single birthday card on his dresser. It read, "To my son, from your father with love." I concluded he and his father were probably close and that I should alert him to the torment I had witnessed. The father's phone number was on an information form I received when Crosby was assigned to me. I knew his father would be in a better position than I was to get major relief for his son.

As soon as I returned home, I phoned his father, introduced myself, and explained my observations regarding his son's pain. He said he had visited his son earlier that day and was aware of how he was suffering. He expressed sadness to see his son go through that. When I asked if he thought that something should be done about the intense pain, he seemed confused about the question. He responded, "What do you mean? I don't think there is anything that can be done at this point. My son is dying, and pain is part of dying." Later that night, Crosby died, probably in pain.

Appropriate pain medication and management procedures must be prescribed by the doctor. After pain medication has been prescribed, it should be evaluated on a regular basis and adjusted as needed. Really listening to feedback of patients regarding their pain is crucial. Treatment for the dying should be done with the same dedication given to cure patients when the goal is to make them well. No one's physical anguish and mental suffering should be left to outmoded, ineffective procedures during the twenty-first century. Patients may need others to advocate for them when their pain is under treated.

A major part of the success in which pain management is done depends on the conditions in which it is provided.

In many nursing homes, much of the actual patient care is implemented by a non-hospice, overworked, changing staff that may need ongoing education in transitioning from a total focus on cure to one of non-curative quality of life. The hospice philosophy of quality end-of-life care should be integrated into the total culture that exists in nursing homes with hospice programs. The nursing home administration should model commitment to this integration, support hospice education for employees, and monitor progress for change to really take place.

A persistent, widespread myth about pain, even among some medical personnel, is that narcotic painkillers such as morphine cause addiction. Another myth is that under treatment of pain during a terminal illness will slow down the death process. There is no truth to these myths when painkillers are monitored properly. Other myths about pain emphasize that it is a natural part of aging and dying, that people who are elderly or mentally unstable can tolerate pain better, that elderly people can't tolerate pain medication well, and that pain medication will make the condition harder to diagnose. Some people believe that patients who don't complain about pain must not have any. Others believe that patients who do complain cannot accurately report their pain. None of these myths is true. That's why it is so important that pain management education be provided for all healthcare workers and the general public.

Patients' pleas for pain relief must be heard and addressed. There are enough types of pain medication available to offer relief to patients. To ignore their pleas is to deny their dignity. They should be asked to rate and describe their pain, even if they don't complain, in case they think having pain is normal. Sometimes patients don't want to bother caregivers with their pain problems. Non-verbal signs of distress such as grimacing, grinding teeth, increased agitation, and sleeping poorly should be viewed as possible pain symptoms. Patients with cognitive or hearing impairment need in-depth methods for pain diagnosis. This could include simplified conversation, pictures, large print, hearing aids, and plenty of patience.

Solutions to the problems of pain management are available now. Nursing homes and other facilities that treat people in pain should keep periodically audited documentation of their procedures. Ineffective pain management, particularly for dying patients with chronic pain, stands in the way of the contentment they should feel at this critical time. While some states are improving in implementing pain management education in healthcare facilities, nationwide progress has been slow.

Jim was the first hospice patient who introduced me to the appearance of real physical pain. Over a series of visits, I learned this lesson well, even after his pain had been reported appropriately. At a personal level, I knew toothaches, sprained ankles, and body-slamming bouts with tonsillitis and the flu. I thought I knew severe pain until I sat in a front-row seat by his bed during several visits.

I watched invisible daggers stab him viciously at sporadic intervals as he lay helplessly. His body tried desperately to curl into an embryonic fist of defense with each attack. Any movement, even breathing, was a bad choice, depending on the timing. Jim's pain was not consistently relieved.

There was no doubt in my mind that a brutal war ensued with pain-free care being the first casualty. Jim was losing the war without his dignity. I was trying to help him fight, but too often, I could only observe and comfort from what seemed like a canyon's distance away. He was in a place I didn't ever want to imagine myself being.

Most days, including after his pain subsided, I seldom understood his words. I questioned him several times about what he wanted me to do for him and paid close attention to his responses, which were usually facial expressions or body movements. Sometimes when he uttered sounds, I gave him water. When he wouldn't drink the water, I started all over again, trying to solve the mystery that would make us both feel satisfied. I knew that finding the solution was my challenge as his volunteer. I grew impatient with myself when I guessed wrong. He was going through so much, I couldn't even begin to be impatient with him.

When I visited Jim, I hoped we would meet mind to mind and resolve our chronic misunderstandings, even if our words were limited. It frustrated me when I couldn't figure out what he wanted. It occurred to me one day that I wasn't sure if I was providing him with anything more than a harder time than he was already having. Did he dread my coming? But my frustration was nothing compared to his suffering. That's what motivated me to keep trying.

In desperation one day, I sat by his bed and held his hand. I noticed that his wrinkled wrist was the size of a child's. I had held his hand many times before, but this time was different. My whole concentration was on non-verbal communication. There had to be another way for me to reach him better than I had been doing. Touch can be a powerful tool. It often speaks a language far better than words.

"It's okay, Jim, I'm here. It's okay," I said to calm him.

"Anne? Anne?" he whispered wearily with his eyes closed, his words moving through teeth like puffs of winter's breath.

His mutterings rose from an exhausted human shell lost in a cave of trauma. But I was sure I had heard him say "Anne." It was the first time I really understood exactly what he meant. I knew that Anne was his deceased wife. They had been married sixty years, and she had been dead five. Still holding his hand, I instinctively became Anne.

I answered, "Yes, Jim. It's me—Anne."

"Help me," he whispered with all his strength pressed into thoughts of hope.

I spoke into his nightmare like I thought Anne would have done, "Jim, I'll always be with you, just like old times when we survived the Great Depression together. You and me, a team forever. We used to have so much fun going places in Detroit. Remember how we used to go to Belle Isle? We'd sit in that beautiful park on sunny days, listen to our favorite music, and watch passing ships. The river flowed like liquid sky. Remember?"

I told him about life in an area of Detroit called Paradise Valley, an entertainment mecca neighboring the Black Bottom residential neighborhood. Negroes prospered there in spite of ongoing struggles against poverty and racism. In that part of Detroit, there were hundreds of Negro-owned places to shop, eat, buy services, and party.

I knew he would remember Paradise Valley because, in those days, it was quite popular. "Paradise Valley was an exciting place, Jim. Blues and jazz hung in the air like comforting fog. Joe Louis, heavyweight-boxing champion of the world, and celebrated writer Langston Hughes walked down those very streets. Oh, and don't let me forget to mention Billie Holliday, Nat King Cole, Duke Ellington, Sammy Davis, Jr., and all the famous entertainers who performed back in the day. They were the best in the country."

I mentioned other popular people, events, and places in Detroit history such as Hitsville USA. That's where inner-city youths like Smokey Robinson and the Miracles, Stevie Wonder, Martha and the Vandellas, the Temptations, and the Supremes were molded into legends. Their music still circles the world with rhythm. I hoped images of the past would help Jim recapture pieces of his life that thrived in Detroit. He created his personal legacy in this city that toughened him to survive his last days in a body racked with distress. I sensed that Jim's mind's eye opened to those blissful memories. For a very brief moment, from somewhere inside the river's horizon, his lips shaped the rarest smile.

The pleasurable spell was broken with another attack from his internal enemies. They had only left to regroup and come back stronger. I started singing "My Girl," an ear-kissing Motown Records song made famous by the popular Temptations singing group. This romantic song sprang from an era Jim could remember when his bed partner was joy, not pain. Maybe years ago, when the sweet medicine of love cured all his sorrow, he had serenaded Anne with the same heartwarming words: "I've got sunshine on a cloudy day. When it's cold outside, I've got the month of May." I hoped the song would be his bulletproof vest that would protect him from an onslaught of hurts.

Once again, he fought his way to a peaceful clearing where he could rest until his next ambush. Sweet memories rewarded him with victory. His breathing relaxed while relief lulled his soul. When he opened his eyes, I was sitting where Anne had been.

Victory

His weary, tucked-in body
lies in a nursing home bed.
A black Gandhi, he yearns for peace.
His days are chains of mountains
formed by pressures of frustration.

I approach him like a helpless child,
wonder how to lift his spirits.
Eyes that have seen ninety years
squint tightly as daggers of pain
pierce his cancerous form.

Intermittent moans of distress
announce his internal battlefield.
A volunteer, I visit him weekly,
try to arm him with weapons
to increase his victories.

Talk, sing, or hold his hand?
Never sure, I try them all.
Words inside he wants to say
are muttered sounds
I seldom understand.

His smile engulfs the room
when I speak of old Detroit.
Perhaps images from the past
recapture stolen pieces
of pleasure from his youth.

I tell him I must leave,
promise to return. Surprising me
in his clearest voice,
he struggles to respond,
"I appreciate your coming."

—Frances Shani Parker

| 5 | Rainbow Smiles | 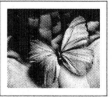 |

Some smiles begin with a warm energy that snakes through your body like a providential python and escapes through doors of your lips. Then there are rainbow smiles that grab you in supersized hugs, hold you so tightly you can feel ribs of joy press against your essence. They are spellbinding, memorable, healing, and enriching, all puckered together in a soul-smacking kiss. Hospice volunteering has been a catalyst for many rainbow smiles in my life. Activities like wheelchair rides, problem-solving, playing games, letter writing, and general conversations are just a few examples of shared time that evolved into celebrations of spirit.

Wheelchair rides brought patients in contact with the world outside their rooms. They provided priceless occasions for me to learn interesting facts about their pasts and their personalities. They gave patients opportunities to extend the boundaries of their experiences beyond their rooms to include other patients, staff, visitors, activities, stimulating sights, and sounds. Hospice provided wheelchairs for its terminally ill patients who needed them.

"See that white line over there?" Gail asks, pointing to a white paint stripe in the parking lot. "That's where I used to park my grey Ford a long time ago. In those days, I was in charge of myself. I could get in my car and drive wherever I wanted to go. I didn't need somebody to drive for me. I just got in my car and started driving. When I built up enough courage, I even went on the freeways and drove out of the state."

"Maybe that's why they call those the good old days, Gail. You had a lot of freedom then, but you can still do interesting things now. You just need a little help to do them. You don't have to have a car to enjoy your life. What I don't understand is how you had a parking spot at this nursing home years ago," I wondered aloud, realizing what she had said.

Sky blue eyes looking upward, she continued, "I lived here in this nursing home on the fifth floor for years. Look up there. That open window on the corner is where my room was. I used to look out that window and see my car. I'd walk around on all the other floors and talk to people. Everybody here knows me, except the new people."

"I'm really surprised. I didn't know any of that, Gail. I thought you moved here recently after you became ill. I guess that makes you a long-time resident of this nursing home. I learned something new about you today."

Talking with patients, I sometimes felt like I was watching them perform a dance of seven veils as they gradually revealed more information about themselves. I was taken aback by her words. It never occurred to me that she had been in the nursing home so many years. I thought she had come after she was diagnosed as a hospice patient. She had a living history there that tapped her on the shoulder, whispered in her ears to remind her of who she had been, what she had done as an independent woman, even as her memory faded.

"Look! The branches on the trees are dancing! And the pretty flowers are all pink, blue, and yellow. They remind me of a big box of pastel-colored crayons. If I could, I'd color all the rooms inside the nursing home these colors. That'd be fun! Then when we woke up in the mornings, we'd think we had fallen asleep out here in the garden under the stars. Take me closer. I want to touch the flowers, feel their softness," Gail requested.

Smiling about the poetic way Gail expressed herself sometimes, I pushed her wheelchair closer to the garden, watched her reach her frail arm out while her eyes reflected nature's pastel bouquet touching her fingertips. I sat on a bench next to her wheelchair, listened to her express every thought that meandered through her mind. Many I had heard before. But time had taught me to be quiet and listen.

When I reached over and held her pasty-colored hand, she smiled and said, "Now that's nice." This simple meeting of skin represented her treasure for the day, week, month, or whatever amount of time had passed since her last encounter with physical affection from another human being. For many patients, these moments seldom came. When they did come, they brought rainbow smiles for sure.

Another patient I had was a dynamo named Nat. He had a large, pancake-sized, cancerous sore covering the front of his neck. Tiny hairs from his beard competed for space in a garden of scabs and bandages that almost always needed to be changed. Getting the bandages changed caused a great deal of pain because particles of scab, dried puss, and hair all came off in the process. More than once, I witnessed him arguing and refusing to cooperate with the nurse trying to change them, even when they were a dirty gray color and looked filthy. Once he threatened to sue anybody who tried to remove his bandages. During those times, he pulled his blanket up to his nose, so no one could see them. Eventually, he would relent and allow the bandages to be changed until the next fight to remove them.

Nat loved his wheelchair rides mainly because they provided him with time for cigarette smoking outdoors on the front porch. Although he had throat cancer, required an oxygen tank next to his bed, and detested having his bandages removed, he never gave up his love for smoking. He enjoyed the cool breeze mixed with smoke brushing against his skin on hot summer days. There was also an indoor smoking area to accommodate him and other patients who wanted to smoke. I held my breath to avoid second-hand smoke every time I briefly entered that room to get a chair. Unfortunately, smoke from the room floated into the halls every time the door opened. In that wing of the nursing home, everybody's nostrils were assaulted with sucker punches of smoke.

Nat's smoking baffled me at first. He knew it was very harmful for him, especially in his deteriorating condition. When I questioned him about it, he said he had tried several times to stop smoking through the years, but he couldn't quit. At this point, he felt it didn't matter. He had spent most of his life smoking, and, according to him, "Everybody dies from something. Why not smoking?"

Hospice is all about providing comfort for patients. A non-smoking volunteer giving lectures on the dangers of smoking to a terminally ill, throat cancer patient isn't very comforting. I let the matter rest in peace. Besides, he had probably heard any lecture I could have given him ten trillion times.

Nat liked to brag about his prowess with women. "You know, I'm kind of a ladies' man. At least, that's what a lot of people have told me. I can't argue with them. I've had a lot of women in my day. Women of all races have found me attractive, including those in foreign countries. I guess I'm like a magnet to them. My problem has always been keeping women around. They never really understand me. Women are complicated creatures. Most of them don't recognize a good man when he's standing right in front of them."

"Did you ever settle down from all your womanizing and get married?" I asked.

"Sure, I got married three times. Each time, I thought I had found the right woman. The first one had a baby with me before we got married. Another baby came later. I had three more kids with my second wife. I didn't have any with my third wife. We got along okay for a few years, but things just didn't work out. Now, she has a new husband who drives my old car that I gave her when I came here."

"How do you feel about that?'

"I don't care. She's a good woman, and she deserves a nice life. We're divorced now, but she still looks out for me, even though I'm in this nursing home. I'm not crazy about her new husband, but we try to get along for her sake. During the holidays, the two of them came to see me. Everything worked out fine, I guess. They took me for a little ride in my car. That was awkward at first, but I was still glad they came. Some people here didn't have anybody take them out. One thing I've learned is that a lot of people are worse off than me."

Nat's ex-wife continued to call and visit him now and then. Several times I pushed him in his wheelchair to the pay telephones in the hall, so he could call her up and talk about how he was doing and what he needed. She always followed through. She was a good woman just like he said.

"Did you see my flag on the side of the bed?" Nat asked me one day.

I looked again at his small American flag taped to the bed railing and responded, "Yes, I noticed it the first day I came. It's always there on your bed. I can tell you like it."

"I fought in a war years ago. Gave the best I could give. I've seen and done things you couldn't imagine. Some of them were horrible, I mean really horrible. Don't ask me to tell you what they were because I can't talk about it. They say time heals all wounds, but it's a lie. I left Viet Nam, but Viet Nam never left me. I carry it with me everywhere I go. All these years later, I still have nightmares like you wouldn't believe. The doctor says it's post-traumatic stress disorder or PTSD. I wake up shaking, gasping for breath with tears in my eyes. In my dreams, I'm always running hard, trying to escape. Sometimes my enemies are close enough for me to touch. I almost stop breathing to keep them from hearing me. I'm constantly thinking I'm not going to make it. Some nights they kill me before I wake up. My dreams are so raw, so real they turn my soul inside out. But in real life, I came back alive. A lot of people who served, some of them my friends, didn't come back. That's why I keep that flag there all the time. It's out of respect for those who came back in bodybags and those still struggling with physical and mental injuries. It's the least I can do for them."

Nat talked to me several times about being released from hospice care. I silently thought his plans to leave seemed unrealistic because his health seemed to be un-raveling more. He felt his health was improving and warned me to call the nursing home and leave a message for him before coming. He said he might be going home any day. I listened to that one-hundred-forty-pound Santa Claus of a man who belonged to my generation, but looked old and ragged enough for a nurse to ask if he were my fa-ther. I knew the day would come when he'd leave hospice care permanently because he was dead. But he wasn't ready to discuss that, so I didn't.

Returning with me to his room from another front-porch smoking excursion, Nat briefly pushed his wheelchair fast to beat the door buzzer that went off when we entered from the porch. This was a race he always won. He never tired of playing this game or bragging about how fast he was every time he won, as if he had hit a home run. People sit-ting in the lobby began to expect that when we entered, there would be a lot of hoopla over Nat's beating the buzzer. The exercise was good for his upper body strength, and he enjoyed celebrating his small conquest.

After we entered the lobby, I pushed his wheelchair through two rooms until we reached the elevator. On the elevator, Nat announced to anyone inclined to listen that I was his wife. That made sense because he had already asked me to make love with him three times that hour. I jokingly threatened to report him to the hospice police if he didn't stop talking like that. Similar to a wheelchair, his mind wove in and out of reality, dodged dangers perceived or real wherever he encountered them.

Like many nursing home residents, Nat shared a room with three other patients. One of his roommates was al-ways out of the room, so I never saw him much. But the other two looked forward to my visits with Nat, so they could marinate in a little attention themselves. Both of them had few visitors.

One roommate was Warren, who was in his sixties and had a throat problem that made his speech difficult to un-derstand. He also walked with a noticeable limp. Grunts, head shaking, body language, and written notes were in-valuable ways he communicated his thoughts. He loved to tease in a playful way that brought out his inner little boy. One of his favorite games was to sneak up behind me in the hall and put his hands over my eyes. Nobody on the face of this earth still did that to me, so I thought it hilari-ous every time he hollered "Who? Who?" to make me guess his identity. He roamed his floor often and greeted every-body. I never knew where I might spot him. When he saw me get off the elevator, he waved frantically and made sounds to get me to notice him. He had definitely mastered the art of making a person feel welcome.

Elvin, Nat's other roommate, was an elderly man who stayed in his room most of the day because he couldn't walk well and didn't feel like making the effort to use his wheelchair. He rarely had a visitor. He liked having a fresh glass of ice water when I gave Nat one. Such a simple act meant so much to him. For several weeks, he didn't say much to me. He seemed confused about my role at the nursing home. Once he mistook me for a nurse aide and told me off for not responding sooner to his call bell. It took me several minutes to convince him he had the wrong woman. Gradually, he began to join in conversations. One day out of nowhere, he announced that he knew who I was and stated my name. Both men accepted that I was Nat's volunteer, but they clearly enjoyed being included. Be-cause Nat had more visitors than they did, he enjoyed sharing our time together as a group.

When all four of us came together in the room, we laughed a lot at one another's eyeball-rolling jokes. Nat and Warren fancied themselves Patients of Comedy, even though their jokes were super corny. When Nat and I teased each other, his roommates joined in our banter, usually taking my side because I was the only woman pre-sent. Before I left from each visit, one of us had said some-thing foolish that triggered four dynamic rainbow smiles that brightened our day. Remembering what Nat had said earlier about women, I was glad to be a complicated creature who could recognize some good men standing right in front of me.

Everyone should be lucky enough to meet a man like Skoney who epitomized "down, but not out." He was in his eighties, a stroke survivor with diabetes so bad that both of his legs had been amputated. When I first saw him, his wide grin hit me like a spotlight. He couldn't speak words at all, and he was blind in one eye. A foul-smelling bedsore or pressure sore on his back needed a machine to drain it. I could see the drainage through a clear plastic tube leading to the machine. It wasn't a pretty sight. With all these problems, he still maintained an optimistic outlook. Fortunately, he had devoted relatives and church members who visited him regularly.

Skoney assumed a "player" persona and flirted with me and other women whenever he could by reaching out for us when we approached his bed. Because his arms were his only limbs for communication, they received quite a workout from grabbing and other motions accompanied by grunting sounds to get his point across. I used to sit by his bed and talk to him, while he used his one good eye to look at me as he processed everything I said. His heart beamed merry messages through that eye that stored more words than a dictionary. Like everyone else, I marveled at his persistence in not being dragged down into life's dungeon of pity, not that anyone would have blamed him. He lit matches of happiness that consumed people with brush fires of delight.

Probably his greatest feat was his ability to outrun the Grim Reaper several times when he came calling for Skoney to leave this earth. But Skoney wasn't ready to go. There were too many things for him to do. He still had more women to reach, more hearts to heal, more love to share, more bright lights to shine in the world. In my mind, even without legs, Skoney was a long-distance Olympic runner who had natural talent for winning survival marathons. He broke records in back-to-back wins on more than one occasion.

People were confused about why Skoney wanted to keep on living with all his limitations. Didn't he know that dying would give him freedom? What was he trying to prove? Because he couldn't talk, Skoney couldn't defend his position, not that he needed to anyway. When he survived each near-death crisis, people shook their heads in disbelief. He received no cheers or back-pats for his outstanding track accomplishments. Observers wondered why he hadn't just surrendered to peace, why he wanted to keep on having comebacks that extended his suffering.

Like any great Olympic runner, Skoney had his own personal-best pace toward his final race. He stayed focused and stuck to his plan, no matter what others said. No one was going to take away his time. Even the Grim Reaper seemed resigned to having races with Skoney. Maybe the two of them enjoyed their private marathons. Clocking more blocks of time in this world was Skoney's choice, even if it meant he would have to struggle more to reach the ultimate finish line

Skoney's last days left him too weak to lift his arms or interact in any visible manner with those in his presence. He had served as an excellent role model for many, particularly those who had serious challenges and needed motivation to keep going. There was a general consensus that, if Skoney could succeed, everyone else could. His love legacy sweetened the air like cinnamon incense. I still crack a rainbow smile when I think about him because, even in death, he grabbed the gold.

Sometimes patients needed me to help them solve problems. One day, Inez and I had an especially great visit. I had been thinking about how to find a key for a music box her niece had given her for Christmas. She loved that music box and liked to have it on display, so she would have a good excuse to talk about it. She had never heard it play because the key was missing when she received it. She said her niece had tried to find a key, but with no success.

The music box was a lovely piece of handiwork. It had a wooden base that supported a clear glass container. Inside the container, lay a beautiful butterfly resting on a small floral bouquet. Underneath the box, was a hidden switch that made the seasonal display enchant with spurts of brightness. Inez, my ninety-two year old patient, said that sometimes she just sat and watched the softly glowing scene quietly blink on and off. One night, she and I silently watched it together. That's when I realized how much this mute little music maker meant to her. Unfortunately, neither of us knew what song it was supposed to play. We imagined the Christmas song we thought it should play and hoped one day we could solve the mystery.

Getting the music box to play became my project, but I knew I would need some help. The next day, I explained the problem to Burton, a teacher at my school. He decided to become a part of the solution by checking out some stores that might have the missing key. It sounded like the search for Cinderella's shoe. After looking for two weeks, Burton finally found a matching key at a large toy store. The sales lady was so touched by his story about Inez's' "musicless" box that she gave him the key free of charge. We couldn't believe our good fortune, which became Inez's thrill maker.

In the second week of May, with spring showing off nature's fashion makeover from winter, Inez heard her cherished, Christmas, music box play for the very first time. She picked it up gently and carefully placed it near her hearing aid. The song we had wondered about for months, the song that had driven us to discover its name finally played. It was a lovely version of "Joy to the World." Just hearing the music box fulfill its purpose felt like a miracle. Inez grinned widely, thanked me, and told me to thank the nice man who found the missing key that made her music box come alive.

The mystery had been solved, and Inez was ecstatic. I thought nothing else that day could outdo the pleasure of hearing the music box play, but I was wrong. After Inez set her mechanical miracle on the window sill, so we could admire it playing and revolving, something wonderful oc-

curred that surprised us both: the brightly colored butterfly started moving, slowing creeping up to the welcoming
red flower. Inez and I gave each other eerie "Twilight Zone"
looks. Then we shared rainbow smiles about the joy in our
own little world.

One of the most challenging patients I ever had, in
terms of finding a creative activity we could share, was
Katherine. She usually lay in bed sleeping or looking up at
the ceiling. Her facial expression was generally neutral. I
couldn't tell if she was bored, unhappy, mellow, or all
three. Pain didn't seem to be a problem. But she couldn't
walk or sit up long, and she rarely spoke. When I first met
her, we mostly stared at each other while I stood over her
and talked. I knew I would have to work hard to find a way
to penetrate the invisible wall between us and then climb
the hill behind it. I felt she was capable of enthusiastic responses, even minimal ones that could saw through the
heavy silence. Not sure she understood anything I said, I
continued to talk to her as if she did, just in case.

I figured the best place to start solving the problem
would be at the beginning. I reviewed the information form
I received from the hospice coordinator when Katherine
was assigned to me. Only very basic information was
given. Among other things, I learned she had come from a
Baptist background, and she was in her nineties. Like
many elderly hospice patients, she had few or no visitors
close to her age. Most of her friends had probably died.

I know that music has a way of melting into parts of our
inner selves, making us feel better when everything else
fails. It occurred to me that Katherine might be able to enjoy some down-home gospel music. I wasn't sure how well
she could hear, particularly above the many sounds that
bombarded her nursing home existence. I wanted her to
have the best musical experience I could provide. That's
when I remembered my CD player that made music meaningful and personal for me when I wore headphones.

With that part of the problem solved, I proceeded to surf
the Internet and research gospel music that was popular

during Katherine's younger adult years. Before long, I found a familiar figure from New Orleans, my hometown. Her name was Mahalia Jackson. Many say she is the greatest gospel singer ever. I remembered hearing Mahalia Jackson's music on the radio when I was growing up. Her records sold multimillions during her forty-five-year career. Thousands paid their respects at her funeral. Among the famous who paid tribute to her were Aretha Franklin and Coretta Scott King. A host of others from all walks of life and various races also came to honor her. Surely, her powerful voice on a CD would inspire Katherine.

I purchased two of Mahalia Jackson's CD's and listened to them just to reassure myself that Mahalia's magic would still work in the 21st century. I wasn't disappointed. Songs like "Didn't It Rain," "When I Wake Up in Glory," and "I'm Going to Live the Life I Sing About in My Song" brought back memories of my own. I headed for the nursing home with what I hoped would be my musical solution. Music would be the bridge. All I needed was for Katherine to cross over.

Katherine lay patiently staring while I adjusted the CD headphones. I centered the headband and placed an earphone on each ear. Her confused expression indicated she had no idea what I was doing. She had probably never seen or heard of a CD player. But with all she didn't know, I sensed she would know good gospel music when she heard it and might even recognize the icon singing. She and Mahalia were all that mattered.

When I turned on the CD player to "When the Saints Go Marching In," Katherine's eyes widened like popped corn. The spirited saints marched in with gusto, rewinding Katherine's mental video to an Alabama church service, urging her to get her praise on. Her hands began to move slowly, and her normally still body jerked slightly. By the time "Little David, Play on Your Harp" came on, Katherine's face wore the best rainbow smile I ever saw.

Sounds of Ecstasy

Headphones frame your head.
You look at me, your volunteer,
wonder what they can be.
Mahalia Jackson's song erupts,
"When the saints go marching in..."
Sleepy eyes widen like popped corn.
"It's a CD player," I say.
Your mental video rewinds
through time—from the nursing home
to an Alabama church service
where bodies rock to music.
I join you clapping with the choir.
Your stiffened hands move
with a powerful energy that rises
like a resurrected hot flash.

"It's wonderful," you whisper.
Mahalia responds singing,
"Walk all over God's heaven..."
I picture you joking with Death
when it's your time to holy dance
to the Other Side of Through.
Mesmerized by the music,
you soak in every song.
A CD player exhilarates you
with sounds of ecstasy.
Such an easy thing for me
to bring, but before I leave,
you say you love me twice.

—Frances Shani Parker

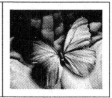
Pointing her out to me, the nurse aide said, "That's Henrietta sitting by herself at the table." I followed her finger to an oatmeal-colored woman who sat humming while folding a napkin. She had just finished eating and still hadn't wiped her mouth. A light coating of chicken grease looked like high-priced lip-gloss when I walked closer to her.

Henrietta was going to be my new patient, my first at this particular nursing home. Later, she would become my first patient whose health improved so much she was discharged from hospice care. For now, she knew nothing about me, including the fact that I was coming. I only knew she was seventy-nine and declining mentally with a form of dementia. I pulled up a chair next to her and said, "Hi, Henrietta. I'm Frances Shani Parker."

Looking me straight in the eyes like she'd known me all her life, she responded, "Girl, I know who you are, long as we've been friends. I've been waiting for you all day. I kept wondering when you were coming. I hoped you hadn't forgotten me, and here you are. What took you so long to get here?"

"Well, actually I got lost," I stammered, processing these new details concerning my whereabouts.

She laughed and said, "Shucks, I get lost all the time. When you get lost, go to the lady at that desk over there. She'll tell you where you are. She'll tell you where you want to go. She knows everything. I'm surprised you didn't go to her before. We all do. How about some dinner? The chicken is something else, nice and tasty, just the way I like it. And I ought to know because I just had a wing that almost made me fly."

"No, thanks. I'm not too hungry now. I'll eat when I go home. Some leftovers are waiting for me. I came to visit you. I want to know if it will be okay with you if I come see you every week."

"Okay with me? Of course, it's okay. Look at all the years you've been coming to see me. If you stopped coming, I'd be wondering where you were just like I did today. So much is on the news, I'd be worried something happened to you. Keep on coming. I don't ever want you to stop."

"I'm looking forward to seeing you, Henrietta. We can talk together, and I can take you on wheelchair rides when I come. We'll get to know each other better, that is, better than we already know each other," I added, remembering our extensive "history."

"Sounds good to me. It's been working for us a long time. I think what you need to do now is eat something. You must be hungry after being lost all that time. Call the waitress over here and order some food. Don't worry about the money. Just put it on my tab. They know me at this restaurant. I eat here a lot."

So, this was Henrietta, an interesting oasis of serendipity. What would the future hold for us as patient and volunteer? I smiled to myself, buckled my mental seatbelt, and prepared for another intriguing ride.

Henrietta was a patient who had dementia, a group of conditions that gradually destroy brain cells and lead to mental decline. Many conditions can cause dementia, but Alzheimer's (Ahlz-high-merz) disease is the leading cause. Most people who have the disease are over sixty-five, with eighty being the average age of diagnosis. According to the Alzheimer's Association, the disease, which advances at different rates, destroys memory and the ability to learn, reason, make judgments, communicate, and perform daily activities. Patients may also experience changes in behavior and personality such as anxiety and delusions. There is no cure for patients with dementia, and eventually they need complete care. The quality of life improves for dementia patients and caregivers when they receive effective care and support.

Working with patients who had dementia introduced me to an interesting world of adult fantasy. Henrietta was one of many patients who kept me on my mental toes when we interacted. Raynell was another. Shortly after Raynell and I met, she started screaming in the middle of our conversation, "Stop it, Robert! Stop it right now!" Then she shook the bedcovers over her feet and yelled to me, "Get him! He's heading under the bed! Hurry before he gets away!" Of course, I was bewildered. Instinctively, I dropped to the floor and started looking under her bed. I thought she might have seen a large spider named Robert. That's how my bloodhound routine of hunting down Robert started.

"Robert, where are you? I know you're hiding under this bed. Show yourself. Speak up like a man!" I pleaded. Thinking about how silly I looked, my inner child grinned at my adult self, a grown woman crawling around looking for a man. After waiting for his silent reply, I pretended he had outsmarted me again with his snakelike quickness.

Robert was an imaginary man who passionately loved Raynell, my eighty-year-old hospice patient. It could be said that he shared a room with Raynell and her three roommates. His presence demanded my attention many days when I went there to visit her. He stole sweetness from the moment by repeatedly pinching Raynell's stout legs. He made her feet rise by pushing up her mattress. Strategically positioned near the foot of her bed, he escaped under it quite easily. That's how Raynell explained the turmoil he caused her. I pulled up a chair in her world each week and made myself at home. While I respected her condition, often letting her take the lead in our discussions, I always remained mindful of my role as volunteer.

Of course, Robert wasn't really the culprit of Raynell's discomfort, which was indisputable. I could see how discolored, sore, and swollen her legs had become with the passage of time. What she was experiencing in her legs was the painful tingling and numbness of nerve damage caused by diabetes, a chronic medical disorder. African-Americans, Hispanics, and several other racial and ethnic groups are more likely to develop diabetes and its complications than Caucasians. While there are genetic reasons for this, environment plays a major role, particularly with Type 2 diabetes, which is linked to diets high in fats and sugars. Raynell had endured this medical disorder for years.

Raynell loved Robert like the devil loves holy water. If she could have cooked him, she would have gladly watched him burst like an overdone potato. He was her personal tormentor. She seemed relieved being able to vent her concerns. I figured Robert was probably locked in a preadolescent love stage and sought Raynell's attention the only way he knew how. Pinching and escaping were so typically boyish. For convenience and his need to be in her airspace, he generally hid under her bed. This worked until I started looking for him when Raynell asked me to make him stop bothering her. Always a step ahead of me, he disappeared as soon as I almost spotted him.

"I wish he would leave me alone," Raynell complained. "I keep telling him I don't have time for a boyfriend. I wouldn't want him, even if I did. I can't tell you how angry he makes me."

"Why do you think Robert keeps hanging around when you've made it so clear you don't want him?" I asked her one day. There was no doubt in my mind that she would have the perfect explanation.

"I don't know what he wants. So far, he doesn't want sex. He's not the one for me. He'll never be the one for me, but I can't make him see that. Last month, I took my foot and kicked him with all my might. I got him good that day. If I ever catch him again, I'll bust his brains out. I mean it. I'm sick of him. You'll never catch him. He's too fast for you, but not for me. One day, I'll get him again just like I did before." I believed her.

Dementia is like a fluttering bee. I never knew when it would make honey or sting. There were times when patients with dementia were rude or violent. I have seen a patient slap a nurse aide's face with such force I thought the aide would fall over. To her credit, the nurse aide took a deep breath and walked away. Another aide interceded. The patient probably forgot the incident soon afterward. During violent situations involving patients with dementia, caregivers had to protect themselves, restrain a patient if they could, but resist expressing rage and fighting back.

Working with mentally challenged patients, I reminded myself that their irrational and unintentional behaviors were manifestations of their diseases. This reminder was similar to the one I used as principal at my school when I dealt with hormonally charged, middle-school students. The vast majority of students behaved very well, but occasionally some were sent to my office for disciplinary problems. Sometimes they were high-strung, defensive, and confused about why they acted out the way they did. Although they rarely admitted it, most students were glad adults stopped their fights. The loudest and most brazen were often easy to reach when no other students were around, and they were more relaxed. Even when their behaviors were intentional, students usually regretted their wrongdoing.

Everybody can't be reached through their front doors. Back doors, side doors, and even windows might be better routes to some people's feelings. The test lies in finding the right entrance through patience, observation, and listening. Similar to some patients, a number of students didn't understand their overreactions and poor choices until they were guided through the right entrance. Viewing behaviors from an impersonal perspective made me and everyone involved calmer, so we could solve problems with less drama.

"You said you played bingo yesterday at the casino. Did you win any of your games?" I asked Raynell. I knew she hadn't left the nursing home to go play bingo at a casino. Because she was often bedridden, she probably had not played bingo at the nursing home either, but she knew bingo was being played somewhere. That was enough to make her an expert bingo player.

"Sure, I win all the time. I'm the bingo queen. Sometimes I do twenty cards at a time to guarantee I have a better chance at winning. But there's something else I need to talk to you about today. It's been on my mind quite a bit lately. I was wondering if you could help me find another apartment. I've been thinking about looking for a new place to stay, maybe a place closer to where I used to live. This apartment building is too noisy. Just close your eyes and listen to all the talking, buzzers, and everything. People come into my place without even knocking. They just walk right in and go through my closet and drawers. It's not right. Three ladies even moved in with me when I wasn't looking. Now, I can't get them out."

"Whoa! That's a surprise! I didn't know you wanted to leave here. Are you sure moving is the best thing to do while you're not feeling well?"

"Lately, I'm feeling much better. I need a change. Even Robert had to leave, so you know it's bad. But I'm very glad about that. He's gone to live in California. I don't think he'll be coming back again."

"A lot sure has happened since I visited you last week. You never said you wanted to move before or that the other people who live here bothered you so much. All this really shocks me."

I thought about this interesting conversation. It was the first time Raynell ever mentioned moving to an apartment and, even more astonishing, the first time she ever said Robert wasn't hiding under her bed. Two weeks later, she was released from hospice care because her health really had improved. She moved to a nursing home near her son's house. I guess Robert knew his time was almost up and decided to leave before he was left.

Patients with dementia communicated with me in ways I found fascinating. Most of our exchanges were good ones. I enjoyed participating as we played mental hide and seek. Occasionally, I buy my inner child festive Mylar balloons that look like flowers, animals, objects, or whatever suits her mood. I take my inner child seriously. Sometimes I'll buy extra balloons for my patients.

"Spring will be coming soon, Miss Robinson. That's a good excuse for me to buy my inner child some Mylar balloons. How would you like a big flowered balloon tied to your bed?" I asked one March day.

"That sounds like fun. I want a balloon, too. Let's see. I want one that's green, all green."

"Really? I thought you might want a pretty flower like the ones on your stationery. I'm getting myself some balloons shaped like flowers."

"No, I don't want a flower. I want a green balloon, just green, no other color. I want all green."

Miss Robinson was very emphatic about choosing a green balloon. She couldn't explain why the color green meant so much to her, except to say it was her favorite color. The party-supply store had many flowered balloons, but green ones were scarce. After a lengthy search with my help, the salesperson found one green balloon in the entire store. Later that week, I brought the balloon to Miss Robinson, tied it to her wheelchair, and took her for an indoor ride around the nursing home to show it off.

"Look, everybody! Look at my red balloon! Did you ever see a red balloon this pretty? It's my red spring balloon! Hey, everybody, look at me! I've got my own red balloon!" she exclaimed.

A few days later, I visited Miss Robinson. Her balloon hovered over her bed like a shiny green pit bull on guard. She could enjoy watching it bobbing around doing its doggie dance and even talk to it if she felt lonely.

"Hi, Miss Robinson. Do you remember who I am?" I asked, giving her a little memory test.

"Of course, I remember you. You're the hat lady who brought me my purple flag. See, it's still waving in the air. I just love my purple flag."

I smiled, thinking of the evolving green balloon that had developed a life of its own. In two weeks, it had evolved at three different levels with hidden powers I hadn't known. It was enough to have gone from a green to red balloon. Now, it had become a purple flag. I couldn't wait to visit Miss Robinson again before the balloon deflated completely. I looked forward to hearing more about the green balloon and its miraculous makeovers.

One of the most spellbinding scenarios that I have witnessed at different nursing homes was parallel conversations among a group of patients with dementia. I have sat at their tables and listened while they took turns speaking about totally different subjects. They looked around at one another and said exactly what was on their minds, often in the most dramatic ways and with no connection at all to what anyone else was saying. One may have been talking about her family, another about a television show, and another about something I couldn't understand. Everything was very pleasant socially, although figuratively no one was on the same street or even in the same town. They fell out laughing at secret jokes that everybody seemed to understand, except me. They had a mysterious dialogue going on that had its own rules. I wasn't sure if mental communication actually took place. I wondered if what they did was similar to how some babies interact with one another. Rather than try to figure it out, I just enjoyed the camaraderie. But I did wish I understood the super funny jokes.

Patients with dementia enjoyed talking and hearing about the past. Frequently, they embellished their stories. Sometimes they remembered detailed incidents from childhood, and minutes later, couldn't remember where they were. They needed encouragement when they became afraid. If they became angry or paranoid, I tried to figure out the reasons why. Distractions helped patients change their thoughts. Just like everyone else, they felt respected when their opinions mattered, so I let them make some decisions, usually limiting the choices to two, so they wouldn't feel overwhelmed.

An important lesson I learned from a patient named Tonya was to accept that I don't know the extent of patients' mental boundaries. Tonya shared a room with one of my hospice patients. I always said, "Good-bye, Tonya" when I passed in front of her bed to go home. I had been doing that for about a year, and Tonya never spoke to me. She looked right through me when I greeted her, as if I wasn't there at all. I knew she was capable of talking, because I had heard her sing and argue enthusiastically with invisible people many times. One night as I was leaving, I said, "Good-bye, Tonya" just like I always did.

"Where are you going?" Tonya asked.

Shocked that she had spoken to me after appearing to ignore me for months, I stared in disbelief and responded, "I'm going home."

"Where do you live?" she continued.

Realizing that she was leading our conversation with sequential statements, proving she understood what she said and meant, showed me how much I had underestimated her mental abilities. I was glad I had continued to speak normally to her in the past when she hadn't answered. Otherwise, our minds would never have met in that moment of enlightenment when the unsaid was said.

"I live right here in Detroit just like you, Tonya."

Focused on my face for the first time, she concluded, "Okay. Go on home in Detroit. Good-bye." She never spoke to me again.

The magnificence of minds, with their startling bursts of thoughts that jar and exhilarate, never ceased to amaze me when I engaged patients who had dementia. Minds that revolved like carousels scooped me up, buckled me in with passion, and carried me on the most fantastic rides. Gatekeepers to an eternal wisdom, they included me in adventures that opened the eyes of my heart, helped me find something I never lost.

With the current state of our world—too often a real-time reality show with high ratings in apathy, greed, and violence—who can say that the world of patients with dementia is worse? Like everyone else, they wrestle with bouts of fear, anger, and sadness. Sometimes their caregivers must dig deeply into wells of themselves for patience and understanding. But who can look through these patients' lens of truth and rate their delusions inferior to insanities in life we say is real? One thing I know for sure is that I visited their Oz weekly and became a better person.

Pieces of Our Minds

On the border, on the brink,
we shiver like quivering tears
swollen to fullness with distress,
reluctant to spill an excess.

Strapped in delusions
wondrous and weird, we ride
roller coasters of reality
through joy and fear.

On the brim, on the rim,
like balls circling in frustration,
we scramble for thoughts
lost in nets of uncertainty.

Invaded by memories,
peeping, creeping, weeping,
we laugh and cry to the
rhythm of nostalgia.

On the fringe, on the edge,
changing, adjusting, impacting,
we crave compassion in our
search for society's sanctuary.

—Frances Shani Parker

7	Love Food	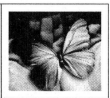

The best love food that can benefit residents in many nursing homes would be more improvements in the general environment. Nourishment is lost when patients are surrounded twenty-four, noisy hours a day by overworked, understaffed, underpaid, and underappreciated workers in an atmosphere of restrictions, schedules, and loneliness. Add to that dying patients with roommates who have varying degrees of physical and mental illnesses. Institutions have unique cultures that impact everyone who enters. When the culture in nursing homes is negative, patients and employees reap negative consequences.

I learned a lot during my interactions with employees. Like any job, there were those who didn't want to be there, but they needed the job. They were resigned to get by doing as little as possible. They resented the work conditions and felt justified holding back on their efforts when they could get away with it. But most of the workers I met appeared to be doing the best they could under trying circumstances. They were often good people who loved their jobs and told me so. There was no hiding the genuine commitment they had made to improve patients' lives. They demonstrated love in their interactions with patients and others daily. What frustrated them wasn't the job, but the game.

Every job has a game that includes the politics, deceptions, manipulations, insanities, and, of course, the stress and energy required to play. Some naïve souls don't realize the game exists, even as they work and complain about matters out of their control. I couldn't help but think how much better employees' and patients' experiences would be if more positive systemic changes took place. More nursing homes should explore ways to enhance their environments with better staffing and training, attractive aesthetics, and innovative procedures for daily routines that reinforce respect for patients and employees.

Zora Neale Hurston, an outstanding American folklorist and writer, stated, "Love makes your soul crawl out from its hiding place." My guess is that she meant this quotation for everybody, especially those close to the end of their lives. Hospice patients need nourishment, a love food with varied ingredients, so their souls can crawl out and know the satisfactions of wholeness.

"Everybody at the senior citizen center asks about you all the time," I read aloud to Jeannine from a letter she had received earlier that week. "We still meet every week to play bridge and gossip. It's not the same without you. People say you were the best bridge player. These days, even I'm winning games. Last week, we had our annual spring party. The last time you came, the two of us ate most of the cookies and didn't feel embarrassed at all (smile). We sure had some good times together."

Jeannine stopped me to explain everything, just in case I hadn't understood what I had read. "See, I learned how to play bridge a long time ago when hardly anybody I knew was playing. My friend Laura taught me because she needed a partner to play with her. I learned as a favor to her and to make new friends. I guess I caught on fast. Next thing I knew, I was teaching her a few things. I remember eating those cookies, too. And they were delicious. We played pranks all the time. We were just a bunch of overgrown kids having a ball cracking jokes whenever we got together."

I observed how animated Jeannine became describing her good times at the center, trying to get me to feel her excitement the way she did. When she allowed me, I continued reading, feeding her a feast of love words. Her friends had taken the time to write her a letter telling her how they were doing and how much they missed her. They signed their names with thoughtful comments next to them, so she would know how much they liked her personally. As I read their names, Jeannine interrupted to mention something special that she remembered about each person. She had gone to the same hairdresser Barbara used, shopped at the grocery with Judy, and first heard about the senior center's bridge games from Laura.

Jeannine had been going to the center for sixteen years. Now, she was in a nursing home away from the buffet of fun they had created. But none of that mattered today. What mattered was that they still cared about her, and she had this cherished letter to prove it. She experienced a mental feast of enjoyment. I smiled, knowing her satisfaction was caused by something she had eaten, something called love food.

Patients were very excited to get mail. Not only did mail bring news from the outside world, it brought affirmations of their worth to others. They wanted their friendship and holiday cards displayed for visitors to notice, pick up, read, and make comments. They were eager to share their written words from others. Of course, letters and cards all received responses that patients dictated to me.

Another way for patients to have positive social contact with people who were not personal caregivers or employees was through recreational activities at the nursing homes. I observed organized activities scheduled and posted at all the nursing homes I visited. Some centers provided an extensive schedule, but others had minimal offerings. Examples of recreational activities were movies, sing-a-longs, bingo, arts and crafts, and entertaining performances. Major holidays were usually celebrated with decorations and a special activity such as a party or dinner. Decorations added a festive quality and reminded residents that a holiday was approaching. During the summer, there were outdoor picnics and barbecues at some nursing home sites.

Patients seemed to benefit from structured activities that improved their skills, morale, and self-esteem. Those who had short attention spans benefited from involvement in projects that reduced boredom, agitation, and their likelihood for having behavior problems. Due to their declining

health, hospice patients were not always able to participate in everything happening, but they were encouraged to
become involved when they could. Social interactions improved their sense of belonging, distracted them from being depressed, and bolstered their independence.
Sometimes they watched from the sidelines while still expressing their opinions and creativity.

"There's a special show going on today in the recreation
room. A group of theater people, you know, actors and ac-
tresses, will be performing a play," I told my patient named
Richard. A pleasant man in his eighties, he rarely remembered who I was, but I knew we connected on some level.

Some days, Richard seemed depressed, as if leaving his
room to spend time with others was too much of a bother.
I focused on ways to help him turn his indifference inside
out and participate in life's fullness, as death's footsteps
quickened down his path. When I heard the theater group
was coming to present a play, I knew that would be a great
activity for uplifting Richard's morale and self-esteem.

"Hmm, people from the theater. What do you think that
will be like?" Richard asked smiling, trying to sort out the
details and maybe warm up to the possibility.

"It said on the flyer they would provide a show with a
variety of acts that would include audience participation.
That means people in the audience can be part of the
show. If you go, Richard, you shouldn't be bored at all.
There will also be prizes and refreshments. I can roll you
there now in your wheelchair if you want to go. What do
you say?"

"I don't know. It might be too much for me. I get tired so
fast, and it could take a long time. I might not even like it.
Would I be back in time for dinner?"

"It shouldn't take too long, Richard. If it's good, you
won't even notice the time. They say time goes by quickly
when you're having fun. If you don't like the show, we can
always leave. I promise to get you back for dinner. I think
it'll be great to do something different"

Richard considered this new opportunity to do something out of the ordinary, still not sure if he wanted to go. Finally, he responded, "I don't know. Maybe I'll just stay here and rest in my room. We can always watch television, maybe one of those shows with the judges. We like to do that sometimes."

"But that's exactly why it would be good to go see this show. Like you said, we can always watch television here in your room. We might not have another chance to see this special performance."

"Is it far away? I'm not up to making a long trip. When I was young, I loved to take trips. But now I'm old. Traveling is too hard. The car could break down or get a flat tire. What would we do then?"

"Where we're going is just down the hall from this room, Richard. We can get there in a few minutes. It's the big blue room where I take you to watch television on days you don't want to go to your room after lunch. Do you remember that big blue room?"

"A big blue room? Is that the room where all the children were one day? They came to sing and play music. I love it when children come to visit. A little boy gave me some cookies and juice. I saw some of my friends there, too. I like that room. Let's go to that big blue room. I remember it now."

Richard surprised me. Instead of associating the room with watching television, he actually remembered another time we had gone there months ago when school children had entertained us. This was another "Whoa!" moment when I remembered his mind's peculiar brilliance. I started pushing his wheelchair before he could find another excuse not to go.

Along the way, Richard greeted other patients and staff members who were headed down the hall in the same direction. Some shuffled along with canes and walkers, while others moved with little or no assistance. Caressing her blanket, a white-haired woman told Richard she was on her way to the airport to catch a plane. A man broke out in song with "We're Off to See the Wizard." I couldn't help rolling my eyes in disbelief when Richard started telling people to hurry, so we wouldn't be late. With each turn of his wheelchair, I could feel his energy growing as we approached the big blue room, a place that made him feel good.

Parking Richard's wheelchair next to a chair where we could sit together, I settled into excitement, glad to have found two good seats near the front. I did another eyeball roll when I overheard Richard proudly tell the man next to him that I was his sister and asked him if we looked alike. Members of the theater group walked in together, enhancing the thrill of anticipation. Their program would be the culmination of hard work. They looked forward to sharing their talents with the larger community, especially with those who might not have the ability or opportunity to come to their public performances.

Exhilaration ignited as the show started. Accompanied by the soft thunder of drumbeats, speakers shared stories and poems in praise of their elders. Patients were given small instruments to play and were coaxed to join in singing lively songs. Dances from back in the day inspired some audience members to sway in their seats. For a soul-stirring while, the nursing home disappeared. We were all transported to a fabulous planet where euphoria was our oxygen. I watched a radiant Richard wave at people he recognized, holler when the emcee gave the signal, and clap like his life depended on it. And the quality of his life really did.

Visitors came in forms besides human ones at a few nursing homes. Animals were great suppliers of love, but I rarely saw any dogs or cats. Animals are allowed in nursing homes in all states. They should be cleared with administrators before they arrive. Anyone who has a pet that would behave appropriately in a nursing home setting can make arrangements to accompany the pet on visits to selected patients. A dog or cat can be tested to become a registered therapy animal. Petting animals can be comforting and therapeutic for patients.

Other animals such as birds and fish have provided a great alternative to the loneliness that became a normal part of too many patients' lives. In the elderly and ill, animals encouraged socialization by becoming topics of conversation that triggered comments and memories from youth. One nursing home had a small aviary with several kinds of birds. Observing the birds interact and listening to their sounds proved to be very satisfying activities. I paused at the aviary to study the birds myself many times before leaving. Watching fish in aquariums, which many of the patients enjoyed doing, was very relaxing, as well as stimulating to their imaginations. Patients wondered how the fish felt and made up stories about how they interpreted their actions.

Because of most animals' non-judgmental acceptance of people, they added a pleasurable component to the nursing home experience in a manner that people couldn't provide. The presence of screened animals at nursing homes was an asset. They entertained, improved morale, and diverted patients' attention away from problems and pain. I felt they were compatible with the nursing home environment because they encouraged stress reduction. In terms of hospice, animals added to patients' quality of life.

Spirituality was another kind of love food in nursing homes. Members of the hospice team did not impose their spiritual views on patients, but they did support patients in their quest for guidance based on patients' beliefs. No matter what their spiritual beliefs were, many patients felt that spiritual counseling helped them make sense out of what was happening to them, grow stronger in facing hardships of their illnesses, and maintain hope for a better future.

Patients were often searching for answers, and some wanted pastoral counseling from their own clergy, the hospice chaplain, or someone who could assist them in exploring their feelings during this critical time in their lives. Knowing that death was impending encouraged some patients to confront issues they might have been avoiding for years. Personal closure in their lives seemed like a proper gesture, particularly when they accepted death and wanted to be prepared to make a good transition. Requested prayers and spiritual readings offered great comfort. Many nursing homes provided religious services, communion, spiritual music, and other materials for those who found solace in them.

Patients usually welcomed visitors of all kinds. Several of my hospice patients spoke about visitors who were not animals or people in the earthly sense. These were deceased family members, friends, and pets. Sometimes visitations were reversed, and patients became the visitors who went to see those who were deceased. I always thought these visits were good signs because wherever the deceased loved ones existed seemed like a wonderful place. When patients were comfortable talking about these visits, I thought it was an indication of their acceptance of death.

Discussions about these visits created opportunities for patients to express emotions openly about death, while reflecting on life. They enjoyed describing their visitors and their trips. Several explained to me in detail, not only whom they saw, but also what the people were wearing. Pets were included in these descriptions. These stories surfaced during normal conversations. One of my patients named Rose, who was almost one hundred years old, enjoyed sharing her experiences.

"What did you do today?" I asked Rose after feeding her.

"Me? I've been spending time with my people. I enjoyed myself a lot."

"Hey, that's great. Did your relatives drive in from Chicago?"

"No, I went to heaven. It's the nicest place, all clean and bright with beautiful sights everywhere. I saw my family and plenty of my friends. They all wore long white gowns."

"Wow! I guess that's a place you'll want to visit again."

"Oh, I'll definitely be going back. I'm planning to go stay there when I die. I'll see if I can help you get in, too."

"Thanks. I would really appreciate that."

"How old did you tell me I was?"

"You're ninety-nine, and you'll be a hundred years old on your next birthday."

"A hundred years old is too old. I don't think I want to be that old."

"There are three other ladies in this nursing home who are older than that. One is a hundred three. We talked to her last week during your wheelchair ride."

"How much longer will it be before I make a hundred? I don't know if I want to wait too much longer."

"It's only one more month. I remember you said you had spiritual talks with your minister. If you decide to wait, I'll get you a big balloon that looks like a birthday cake."

"I guess I could wait. Yes, I think I will wait. That way I can celebrate my hundredth birthday. When I do get to heaven, I can tell everybody I lived to be one hundred."

And that's exactly what she did.

Missing

She waited,
hoping her years of caring
endured in grown-up minds,
rested in distant hearts,
conveyed how much she missed them.

She waited,
living real-time movies
of restless nights, anxious days
with inhaled hopes of fellowship,
exhaled sighs of deep despair.

She waited,
wishing nostalgic winds
flowed through cotton curtains,
brought relatives and friends
she cherished through the years.

She waited,
grasping like a New Year's resolution,
like a second suspended in time
until her clock stopped ticking
for visitors who never came.

—Frances Shani Parker

8	# Mealtime Gathering	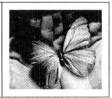

I sat waiting for meals to arrive in the third floor dining area. Having performed this ritual at many nursing homes, I knew the drill well. Patients dribbled in moving slowly, many using canes and walkers. Others arrived in wheelchairs that twisted and turned as they parked in chosen spaces. Mentally competent residents tended to congregate together. However, they did look out for those patients with dementia who had nowhere else to sit except with them. Most patients didn't seem to mind where they sat. Those who could maneuver themselves mentally and physically on the elevators often went to the main dining room on the first floor to eat. But those in need of supervision and assistance remained on their own floors.

Meals were delivered via the elevators which stopped at dining areas on four other floors. The fish in the aquarium probably slapped fins and laughed as they watched us complain impatiently about waiting. This must be how they felt when they checked for floating food while waiting for busy humans to feed them. Maybe that's why they found us so amusing as we watched slow-moving clock hands and elevator doors that seldom opened. Elevators were slow anyway, but, at mealtimes, they moved like arthritic turtles. It's a long process, but it's best to report on time and be seated, just in case we were surprised, as we were occasionally, with meals arriving on time.

Some weekend employees who were not regular members of the staff appeared to be less skilled in certain procedures. I often scheduled my visits during times when meals were served, so I could give my assigned patients more attention when nurse aides were very busy. I had noticed that conversations with patients were often engaging when food and socializing were combined. Several of my patients had not been able to feed themselves, but my current patient only needed a little assistance.

Although I went to the nursing home primarily to serve patients assigned to me, it was impossible to isolate meal-time visits with my patients from the rest of the nursing home community. From the time I entered the building, I found myself in a humming hive of employees, visitors, and other patients. Feeding my own patients was viewed as helpful to nurse aides because it reduced the number of patients they would have to feed themselves. Over a period of time, they had come to know my purpose for being there and seemed glad to see me.

More waiting took place after the large food carts arrived. I helped out sometimes by putting bibs on all the patients. Clearly, more help was needed, especially on very understaffed days. Each patient's labeled tray had to be found and distributed. Coffee had to be poured with optional cream and sugar added. Salt, pepper, salad dressing, butter, ketchup, mustard, and mayonnaise needed to be added to entrees that often had to be cut into smaller pieces. Mealtime at nursing homes was no small feat, particularly when many patients needed to be individually fed or assisted.

Today, I convinced my patient Naomi to join others in the dining area instead of eating in her room. She usually liked to join them, but today she wasn't sure if that was the right thing to do. She asked anyone, "Am I doing the right thing?" Naomi wanted to be a good person, and everybody who associated with her said that she was. I pushed her in her wheelchair to the dining area and assessed the situation. I targeted a table with an empty space that looked big enough for her wheelchair to fit and for me to sit next to her. The spot I found, in which I shoehorned both of us, was located at a table for eight. I was the only person at the table without dementia. While my focus was on assisting Naomi, I knew I would probably have to supervise, encourage, and generally keep an eye on everybody at the table. The nurse aides would be too busy feeding patients at their own tables. When seven patients with dementia get together to eat at the same table, all kinds of scenarios can occur. I instinctively went into multitask mode.

"This tray has your name on it, Naomi. All this food is for you," I said to Naomi, who was in her nineties. I had stood near the carts, so the aides could hand me Naomi's tray to fix as soon as they found it. Sighing deeply, one aide told me, "Thank God you're here today to help." I knew exactly how to fix Naomi's tray. She liked her coffee hot and black. She preferred drinking cold liquids from a straw. She wanted all the condiments. I left her wrapped bread on the tray, but I knew she wouldn't eat any. Naomi was a good eater until she saw ice cream. She absolutely adored ice cream. The aides and I knew that if Naomi saw her ice cream cup, she would eat her ice cream first and ignore the rest of the meal. She did this, not because she wasn't still hungry, but because she wanted more ice cream to satisfy her hunger. Naomi would probably eat ice cream all day if she could. I put her ice cream cup on the side where she couldn't see it, so she could eat it later.

"Look at what you have here to eat, Naomi—coffee, juice, milk, mashed potatoes, fish, broccoli, bread, and fruit. That's a lot of food. It looks good. Try some. Tell me what it is and how you like it." Naomi looked over her plate, took a spoonful, and did an evaluation. "I think everything looks good. But my ice cream tastes funny. I don't like it like this," she complained after chewing the mashed potatoes.

"That's because it's not ice cream, Naomi. Those are your potatoes. I'll see if I can find some ice cream for you after you eat a little. Try something else and tell me what you think it is."

"Okay," Naomi responded as she began to eat her fish and told me what it was. When she took a sip of coffee, I already knew she would say, "Mmmmmm good. Nice and hot!" I laughed when she did this, because my prediction was right again, but I didn't tell her that.

Some patients were confused about which utensils to use. They tried to eat soup with a fork if they were not guided to a spoon. For a few, the tray of food was more like a tray of colors that smelled like food. Sometimes with pureed food, they had no idea what they were eating, and neither did I. Fortunately, a menu came with each tray. At one nursing home, I observed a nurse aide telling a blind patient everything on his plate when she sat his tray in front of him. He grinned with delight the whole time she went down the list of foods. That's why I started telling my patients what was on their plates. Even those who could see didn't always know what was there.

I continued talking to Naomi and assisting her while monitoring others at the table. I noticed that Petra had not touched anything. Petra was not a very independent eater, but I knew she was physically capable of feeding herself by any means necessary.

"Petra, your food is just sitting there getting cold. You have a whole tray of delicious things to eat. You should eat some and see how good it is. You're a good eater. Eat your food."

"Food? What food? I don't have none."

"The food on this tray is all for you, Petra. This is your food tray right in front of you. Watch me point to each item. You have coffee, juice, milk, mashed potatoes, fish, broccoli, bread, and fruit. That's your name spelled P-e-t-r-a."

"That's not my name. My name is Petra. That's somebody else's name. That's not my name. I know my name."

"Well, that is still your food on the tray. You should eat before it gets cold. Go ahead and eat. Give it a try."

"Eat? Eat what?"

"Your food, Petra, your fish, potatoes, and everything else."

"Fish? What fish? I don't have none. Do you see a fish here? I don't see a fish. I don't have none."

From previous experience, I knew that Petra and I could go on roaming forever around this same circle. Luckily, she was sitting next to me. I gave her a taste of the fish because I knew she liked it. Then I placed her fork in her hand and started her off eating. I did this in steps by steering her hand and giving her directions on putting food into her mouth, chewing, and swallowing. Patients with dementia needed tasks broken into simple steps. Usually, she ate for a while by herself, even with her hands, once somebody started her off. Without any help, she sat and looked at the food she said was not there. My other hand continued to assist Naomi.

"Don't do that! Leave my food alone! Get your nasty hands off my plate! Help! Can somebody help me?" screamed a patient at our table as if she were under attack. All the nurse aides were occupied feeding patients at other tables and experiencing their own mealtime problems. I was resigned to be the unofficial table captain now. I told Roscoe sternly to leave Charlena's food alone. He gave me a confused look, pretended he didn't know what I was talking about, but betrayed himself with a silly smirk he thought I didn't see. I leaned across the table and directed his attention to his own plate by putting his spoon in his food. He picked up his spoon and started eating again. Then I reassured Charlena that everything was okay, and she could finish eating. Charlena smiled with an air of triumph. Roscoe was in trouble, and she relished knowing she helped to get him there.

Rita had been watching me help Naomi and Petra eat. Now, she was attempting to feed George, but with her own used utensils. George had his mouth open obligingly, anything to help the cause. I interceded before any damage was done. By this time, several patients had spilled food on the table or the floor and had food stains on their bibs. Petra had to be restarted twice to eat the food she insisted she'd never received. I had stood to lean across the table three more times to settle other table disputes involving food and different patients.

Naomi ate right along during all the interruptions. I had been giving her ongoing praise on how well she was doing. I also praised others at the table when they did well. They savored the attention, and Naomi wasn't the least bit jealous. She had already told the others that I was her guest and offered me food, which I declined. I hadn't gone there to eat and couldn't even think about eating if I had. When one patient was praised, another would often say, "Look at me. I'm eating too." This reminded me of students at my school. They said the same thing when someone else was praised. I laughed, thinking the world was a universal classroom. Maybe the stars in the sky were created to be placed on billions of people's foreheads when they did something praiseworthy.

At the next table, I noticed a caregiving husband feeding his wife. She drooled uncontrollably, and he used one hand to assist her with eating and the other to continuously wipe her mouth. He had brought some food from home to supplement the nursing home meal. The sweet potato pie distracted a few patients who wondered why they didn't have any. The husband had told me earlier that he hadn't felt well lately. I reminded him to be sure to take care of his health, so he could keep on being a good caregiver to his wife. I knew that the percentage of dementia sufferers who outlived their caregivers was increasing. Caregivers should never neglect their own health.

A daughter fed her mother who sat in her wheelchair near the dining area entrance. Every day the daughter or her brother came with food made especially for their mother. The mother couldn't talk, but she did make facial expressions and nod to give her daughter feedback on how she was doing. She ate well and loved this personal attention. The daughter and brother were good advocates, always checking and making corrections to improve their mother's care when necessary.

At another table, a man sang a spiritual song loudly through most of the meal. His voice was deep, rough, and confident. In another setting, without a television playing in the background and mischievous, caffeine-drinking diners who didn't need much to get hyped up, he might have been applauded. Several aides asked him to be quiet, and he stopped periodically. But as soon as the spirit hit him again, he broke out in song with or without a choir director's permission.

One patient started "cleaning up" her table by scraping others' leftover food on one plate. The receiving plate, which looked like a Frisbee-shaped dumpster, was placed in the center of the table. Leftover scraps were piling up fast. Hopefully, she had a backup plan for the overflow. This was not her job or anyone else's at the tables, but unless the other plates were removed from her table right away, she always assumed this role. Another woman had to be reminded several times to stop raising up her dress and exposing her diaper. She talked back and cursed at the aide who corrected her. A man who smiled contently after eating his meal was told to take his hand out of the front of his pants.

Naomi was almost finished. She'd eaten well from each food group and asked about her ice cream several times. I watched her beam like a prom queen when I told her what a great job she'd done. I handed her the ice cream cup. She became ecstatic with joy and squealed, "My ice cream! My ice cream! You found my ice cream!" After she took her first swallow, I asked her about the flavor, the color, the coldness, and, of course, the taste. Ice cream eating was serious business, and Naomi was a connoisseur. She described everything in detail between spoonfuls that she ate slowly. I never knew anybody could love ice cream the way Naomi did.

A few patients who finished early were starting to nod off into their naps. Mealtime was usually followed by time socializing or resting. Some patients sat around watching television shows or videos. Others used this time to talk to themselves, have parallel conversations, or talk to one another. Compatible roommates enjoyed teasing one another after eating. They told me the funniest stories while mocking one another, but their mutual friendship was always evident. One lady jokingly threatened her roommate by balling up her fists saying, "Girl, if you wake me up one more time, I'm going to knock you into next week." Responding in a gruff tone and balling up her own fists, the roommate hollered back, "Bring it!" Both women were in wheelchairs.

Some people preferred rolling their wheelchairs back to their rooms right away. They'd had enough socializing during mealtime. Aaron liked to put his head on his folded arms on the table and take a nap until an aide took him to his room. Pat was perfectly content folding napkins and bibs over and over. I imagined she was a dedicated scientist looking for the perfect shape, and there was no hurry at all. The world would have to wait for her earth-shaking discovery, just like we waited for food to arrive on our floor.

Mealtime had come and gone. Patients were fed and quieter now. Later, the dining area would be cleaned for the next mealtime gathering. Patients were taken to use bathrooms or get diapers changed in preparation for the rest of the day or nighttime. Naomi invited me to come back and be her guest again at another mealtime. I told her I would return the following week. Before I stepped on the elevator to leave, she looked at me innocently and asked, "Did I ever tell you I love ice cream?"

Mealtime Party

"Come to your party, Lurania! Have some tacos!
We're singing in Spanish!" Lurania exclaims.
Her two-part conversations go back
and forth like a tennis match with one player.
Today, Lurania gives someone else her name,
so she can host an imaginary party for herself.

Next to Lurania sits sleeping Mary.
A purring snore drifts from her open mouth,
a canon too tired to fire. All morning,
she searched for her slippers
until she found them on her feet.
Now, she salsas in her dreams.

"10, 9, 8, 7, 6, 5..." yells John, who thinks
Lurania's party is on New Year's Eve.
He holds up his milk carton and shouts,
"Happy New Year!" John knows
the wish everyone wants to hear
as 12:00 noon begins another year.

Grace still wears the glow of a woman
who's been in love. Her so-called boyfriend,
a nurse aide sixty years her junior,
blushed when told of her romantic fantasy.
Even though she "dumped" him,
their friendship will be a lasting flower.

"You know, Olga has been my sister
all my life," Miller announces. I remind him
that yesterday Olga brought him
a chocolate chip cookie. Miller flaunts
a grin, satisfied that the streetcar
of his life looks great, rides just fine.

"Everybody can come! Lurania's parties
are wonderful!" Lurania hollers, intoxicated
with laughter resonating like a trumpet.
Everyone should come and marvel
at the magnificence of minds that dance,
turn somersaults to create happy realities.

—Frances Shani Parker

9	# Death ## Sentences	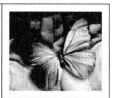

As sure as rain escorts a hurricane on a turbulent date, cosmic harmony mandates that each person arrive on the Other Side of Through. Death will come, no matter how often the topic is avoided, how forcefully technology wrestles it to the ground, how clearly pleas for more earthly time are heard. People will be confronted with their mortality whether they like it or not. Those who listen to the universe will be reminded to squeeze out all the pleasure they can in life, give service to others, and drink blessings with gratitude.

Comments about death would not be complete without an acknowledgment of possible life after death. Many people believe in life after death. For them, death is a comma, a pause proceeded by a dash into another dimension of life. Others say that life, as we know it while living, is all there is to existence. They consider death to be a period at the end of the final sentence in their life stories.

One day, I had an interesting conversation about life after death with my patient named Mabel. Previous to this conversation, she had refused to discuss anything related to death, including the death of one of her roommates. She said her roommate had to be carried out a few days earlier and was gone for good. Shaking her head sadly, she changed the subject. We both knew her roommate had died, but she couldn't bring herself to say that word. Although hospice team members never impose religion on patients, Mabel decided to explain her religious views to me anyway.

"This is a lovely birthday card from some of your church members," I commented, admiring some recent birthday cards Mabel had received. The cards formed a cheery conga line along the windowsill.

"Yes, that was nice of them to remember me and send me cards," she said, "I've been going to that church quite a few years. They keep a directory of everybody's birthdays. Even though I don't attend church there now, they still remember my birthday."

"Were you active in your church?"

"Well, not too much. I helped out with a few fundraising activities like the annual church bazaar. I usually worked at the ticket booth. I didn't want to be too active because I have my own personal views about religion. I don't see religion the way most of my church people see it, so I stayed kind of low key. Religion is fine, but I don't believe in God. I only believe in Jesus."

"Really? Why is that?"

"Jesus was a person in real life. People saw him and wrote down what he did and what he said as part of history. I know that Jesus existed. He was right there walking and talking in front of people. Nobody can deny that. But God is different. Nobody has really seen him. Nobody knows how he looks or even what he is. That's why I don't believe in God. But I definitely believe in my Jesus."

"What about heaven? What do you think of that?"

"If there is no God, then there is no heaven. It wouldn't make sense to have a heaven without God. That's how I see it."

"What do you think happens after people die?"

"What do I think happens? Nothing. They get buried, and their problems are over. Their problems end, and ours continue."

Mabel's belief about life after death was one of numerous opinions that people have. Many have thought about the possibility of immortality. They connect it with a soul, reward, and punishment. Some have lived their lives according to those beliefs. For those who believe in an afterlife, there is often a spiritual motivation linked with nature's cycles of birth and death. They embrace the mystery with faith and decide there is no spiritual death, only a change in their immortal soul's experience.

Of course, a lot of people say they don't know what to believe. Scientific research on near-death experiences and other death-related phenomena continues to accumulate data to shed new light on discussions about life after death. Ultimately, people have to decide for themselves what they want to believe.

"Tell me about your life when you were growing up, Jackie," I said to one of my Caucasian patients. I was recording her life review, a written legacy that would be put in booklet form for her family and friends to treasure after her death. It could also be made into a CD or a video. Many hospice patients enjoyed creating this record, adding permanence to their history. Jackie was glad she could still remember what had happened in her life and eager to tell me her story. She had been thinking about her life because she knew I would be asking her questions. Memories she shared would be significant in showing who she was and why her life mattered. She was glad she felt physically strong enough to discuss her life for several visits with me until her life review was finished.

Jackie explained, "There's really not a whole lot to say. I had two parents, a brother, and a sister. We lived in a rural area in Ohio. We didn't have much money, but we were always clean and fed. We hardly ever got sick. My mother was a good cook. She taught me how to cook all kinds of foods. My specialty was pies. I made the best lemon meringue pies you ever tasted. That's what everybody said. Making a pie every week gave me a lot of practice."

"I sure wish we could eat one now. What did you do when you wanted to have fun? Where did you go when you left the house?"

"There wasn't much to do for fun. We all had chores that had to be done by a certain time each day. My job was mostly helping with the cooking and cleaning inside. We played ball and jumped rope outside. During the week, we went to school. The whole family went to church on Sundays. Going to church and studying the Bible were important. When the holidays came, we all went to visit relatives who lived in the next town. Holidays were always happy times for us."

"What were your dreams about your future? As a young girl, did you have dreams you wanted to achieve that motivated you? Did you have something that you really wanted to accomplish in your life?"

"Oh, I had lots of dreams. I wanted to be an actress, hear the sounds of people's hands clapping just for me. I used to listen to plays on the radio, close my eyes, and pretend I was standing on a stage somewhere saying my lines. I wanted to travel all over the world and see what life was like in places I read about in books. I thought it would be great to learn another language and use it later to speak to foreigners, especially if I traveled somewhere. I never got to do all that, but I did learn a little French and finished high school. I married my first boyfriend and had three children, just like my mother did."

"Did you have any close friends?"

"I had a few good friends. The one I'm thinking about now was a colored girl about your color. Her name was Oni. I liked her a lot. But when I told my mother about her, she said I could be Oni's friend, but to never let her come to our house. She also warned me not to talk about her when my father was around. She told my sister and brother the same thing. When I asked her why, she said my father didn't like colored people, and he wouldn't like it if he knew I was friendly with one. I was shocked to hear that, especially since we went to church and read the Bible and all. I had no idea that my father didn't like colored people. He never said he didn't. After I thought about it, I realized there weren't too many colored people around where we lived. None had been to our house, except to do some work. We all agreed to keep the secret about my colored friend from my father."

"What was that like, having a friend you cared about and having to keep her a secret because of her race?"

"I didn't like it at all and neither did Oni. I guess my father was a racist. He didn't even know Oni, but he had already judged her in the wrong way, just because of her race. I wish he could have seen what a good person she was. The strange part was that he didn't realize he was racist. Even though Oni and I were children, we knew we wouldn't let my father's feelings about race come between us. We played together whenever we could. We shared secrets and helped each other out. I could tell her anything, and she was really smart about figuring things out. My mother wasn't like my father. She didn't want to get him upset, so she never told him he was wrong. She told us children that we should be open to knowing all kinds of people and love everybody the way the Bible says we should. I'm just glad my mother told me what was right. If she hadn't, I would have missed out on knowing the best friend I ever had."

Truth has a sourness to it that many don't want to taste. They avoid it, convince themselves that they are justified, even when no rational reason can defend their unwillingness to sample all that truth has to offer. But tasting is the only way to distinguish its unique mix of flavors, to savor its bitter sweetness, to swallow with unexpected satisfaction. Discovering that satisfaction makes those who shun truth wonder why they ever resisted.

Assumptions should never be made about all people who belong to a particular group. A volunteer should keep in mind that people in a particular racial, ethnic, or religious group may not all share the same customs and values. The best way to respond to families regarding their customs and values is to ask them. Death rituals usually evolve from religious, cultural, and traditional beliefs. Having a degree of familiarity with different death rituals in America gives the volunteer an advantage in being sensitive to families' needs. For example, in the Christian tradition, family hours with viewing of the body often precede funerals. However, the Jewish death ritual does not display the body publicly.

Many African Americans have strong religious views about death being equated with going home. Releasing emotions freely at wakes and funerals is acceptable as a means of coping with loss and celebrating the journey home. As a child raised in New Orleans during the Jim Crow era of racial segregation, I remember attending several night wakes, viewings, and family hours at "colored" funeral homes where bodies were on display. A casket was usually opened, so those who came to pay their respects could walk up, view the deceased, and say a silent prayer. This was done slowly with awareness that others in the room might be watching their responses to viewing the body. Viewers read the cards attached to flowers displayed near the casket. Before being seated, they extended condolences to immediate family members, who usually sat in the front rows. Families appreciated support from the community.

Viewers sat in rows of chairs facing the casket and softly talked among themselves. This time together was a reunion for them as well as a time to discuss how the body was dressed and "fixed up" with cosmetics. Comments about the deceased wearing a smile, looking peaceful, or appearing to be asleep were considered good compliments. Once I heard that a woman said the deceased "must be hot in that winter suit" during a wake held in July. Everybody wanted to believe that the deceased was content, especially if there had been suffering before the death. A brief service was held. There were concerns about how the family was "taking it," along with lots of reassurances that there was no need to worry because everything was in God's hands and would be all right.

I looked forward to going to wakes, not because I found them entertaining, but because I appreciated the seriousness and empathy of the rituals. I never experienced fear being close to open caskets. In my child's mind, the "real" dead people, the ones I actually knew, were in heaven somewhere, and their harmless bodies had been left in the caskets as reminders for us.

Next to viewing bodies, my most memorable experiences at wakes centered on eating refreshments served in another room at the funeral home. I loved the chicken salad sandwiches cut into triangular shapes without crusts. We wouldn't even think of removing bread crusts at home. Those sandwiches were rare treats, and I still love chicken salad sandwiches. My attendance at wakes, funerals, and other rituals taught me to respect rituals in general. Nowadays, I enjoy creating my own rituals.

I have attended several funerals in my role as hospice volunteer. Most were traditional Christian funerals where I met many family members and friends of deceased patients for the first time. I learned new information about my deceased patients. Expressions of gratitude for caring services of the hospice team often sprinkled conversations. One especially nice funeral concluded with an announcement inviting everyone in the church to lunch at a popular Detroit restaurant. Sharing food and stories with relatives and friends brought perfect closure to my hospice experience with that patient.

Sometimes, however, hospice patients died without a supportive family or financial accommodations for death rituals. For many of them, loneliness had replaced oxygen throughout their illnesses preceding death. Some were dispirited about life in general. Such was the case with Lelia. When I first met her, she was sitting alone in a dimly lit room she shared with three other women. Her blouse was unbuttoned, exposing one sagging brown breast and a wormlike scar where her other breast had been removed. Depression embraced her like a close friend. A wary look in her eyes told me she had no place for a hospice volunteer on her agenda.

"What's that, you say you a hospice volunteer and you want to come see me every week? No, I don't need to see you. I have enough visitors," Lelia complained shortly after I arrived. Her tone reeked with annoyance at my intrusive presence in her gated world.

"Lelia, I came by to see you today because I hoped we could get to know each other better. I was thinking that I might be able to help you in some way, maybe with a problem or something."

"No, I got enough help. Like I said, I don't need to see you. I don't need to see nobody. I just want to be left alone."

"Okay, if that's what you want, then I won't come back. I notice you have a candy bar on your table. Is that your favorite kind?"

"No, somebody just brought that here and left it there. I never told them I wanted it. Some people think they know what I want better than I do. My favorite candy is Tootsie Roll, but nobody brings me that. I don't care. I don't care about nothing."

"Well, I guess I'll go now. No point in hanging around taking up your time. It was nice meeting you, Lelia. Too bad we won't see each other again. But I can understand if you already have enough visitors. I would have brought you some Tootsie Rolls when I came back, but now I don't have to worry about doing that," I said, standing up, turning to leave.

"You leaving now? How come you in such a hurry? You already here. Maybe I could use a little company just for right now. Look, you don't know me. I got problems, big problems. I can't trust nobody, not even my own family."

"Tell me about your problems. I'll just sit here and listen. Then we can talk about what you said. If we don't get finished discussing your problems today, we can finish next week when I come back with Tootsie Rolls. What do you think about that?"

"I think I could deal with that. You say you coming back next week with some Tootsie Rolls? I like the little ones. You won't forget will you?"

"Forget you and your Tootsie Rolls? I don't think so."

After that first day, Lelia and I looked forward to talking every week. Her life book included many heartbreaking chapters. She told me about her younger days struggling in a touring singing group. Later, her husband and four children drifted away from her life and one another. She explained her agonizing breast cancer and the injustice of all that had happened to her.

Lelia was a hammer looking for a nail. She had grown paranoid of others and was especially upset about her sister Essie, who had put her in the nursing home. She felt that Essie was getting all her money and spending it without her consent. It bothered her that somebody else could spend her money like that. Helpless to do anything about life's perceived or real injustices, Lelia resigned herself to mental misery.

But some days, she glowed with gladness when a few good times she had experienced in life slow-danced into her wavering memory and made her eyes sparkle. With no teeth at all, she managed to suck the entire flavor from the small Tootsie Rolls I brought. I watched in amazement as she relished each chocolate-flavored morsel with gourmet gusto worthy of a Super Bowl television commercial. Unfortunately, her health continued to roll downhill like a battered ball. One day, I received the hospice phone call saying she had died.

The hospice organization provided the ritual that commemorated Lelia's death. A small group gathered in the recreation room at the nursing home. Most people present were other patients who knew Lelia. Essie, Lelia's sister, came with a friend named Nola. The hospice chaplain opened the memorial ceremony with a prayer and a reading. Taking turns, we shared our memories of Lelia. Some comments were hilarious, while others revealed Lelia's demons. We all discovered new layers of Lelia that came together in a mental mural of colorful qualities.

Essie spoke last, "I'm sitting here in shock listening to what you all said about my sister. I can't believe we knew the same person. The Lelia I knew hardly ever said anything funny, and she sure wasn't thoughtful, at least not to me. Even when I helped her get into this nursing home, she still acted like she hated me. She was grouchy and liked to criticize people all the time. Nobody was really close to her. To tell you the truth, nobody in our family was close to anybody else in the family. There was just too much drama going on all the time. That's why I'm the only one here. I started not to come myself, but now I'm glad I did. I learned something new today. I feel better about Lelia after hearing your stories."

Although the chaplain hadn't known in advance how many would attend the ceremony, she had brought twelve helium balloons, the exact number needed for each person present to have a balloon to release later. Swaying like colorful hula dancers, from strings tied to a chair, the balloons added a festive energy to Lelia's homegoing. Riding down with the group on the elevator, Nola mentioned that she and Essie were singers. We all agreed they should lead us in song when the balloons were released during our tribute to Lelia.

Our humble circle stood in the front yard of a Detroit nursing home to perform our final death ritual for Lelia. People riding by in cars on a busy street observed a lively group of ecstatic mourners looking upward, enthusiastically singing "Going to Shout All Over God's Heaven." Passionate voices resonated like rockets. We released our buoyant balls of bliss floating in a hurry to get somewhere. I imagined Lelia looking on, bobbing her head to the gospel beat. She grinned her toothless rainbow smile that colored our hearts with joy from the Other Side of Through when we all yelled, "Bye, Lelia! Have yourself a good time!"

The Other Side of Through

Another world awaits you
where land and sky embrace.
Spirit, wisdom, nature
celebrate your arrival.
Journey where sounds
vibrate with peace,
rain splatters blessings,
language flows into every heart.
What fun it is to swim
in rivers of conversations
kept afloat by mutual goodwill
when everyone clings
to rafts of one another.

Feast at tables where
hunger can't be remembered,
kindness is never forgotten,
laughter tickles the universe.
Let your fertile mind
grow bouquets of ideas,
silence hold you in its arms
while the unsaid is said.
Live miracles every moment
with worry-free days.
Time has no reason to fly,
no way to be wasted,
no wounds to heal.
Can you feel the love?

—Frances Shani Parker

Part II:

Footsteps to Caregiving, Death, and the Future of Hospice

10 Caregiver Guidance

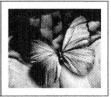

I have witnessed or participated in interactions between patients' family members and friends on many occasions. Their involvement as caregivers added immensely to the progress of patients emotionally, spirituality, socially, and physically. This was especially true when close bonds already existed. Caring relationships eased stressful situations that caused barriers to support and communication. In cases where bonds were unglued long before patients became residents in nursing homes, difficulties that arose were sometimes harder to negotiate and resolve, but not always. A lot depended on the nature of the problems, the people involved, and commitments to relationships.

Ongoing presence of family and friends impacted the quality of care and ultimately the quality of patients' lives. Families tended to prefer that their loved ones were at home instead of in nursing homes. But they could no longer meet their needs at home anymore. Patients sometimes preferred to be at home, even when they knew they were dying and needed more care than they could receive there.

Adjusting to nursing home life was not always an easy process for caregivers or patients. Being placed in a nursing home gave patients a feeling of hopelessness and loss. They were often totally dependent on others to fulfill their basic needs. Some patients were depressed about having to give up so much of what had belonged to them for most of their lives. Although they may have understood rationally that there had been no other choice, they expressed their resentment toward relatives for putting them there. There were patients who had no idea what was happening to them. They only knew that their lives had changed drastically with different people, sounds, and scenery. Nothing was familiar anymore. Confusion reigned. Sometimes life seemed overwhelming. Family members often felt guilty about patients, who had loved and taken care of them in earlier years, being taken out of their homes. But home care was no longer safe for patients who were a danger to themselves and others. Some patients' resentment towards being in a nursing home extended to a bitterness directed at employees and visitors. This embarrassed family members and made the adjustment to a nursing home setting even more difficult.

Patients were not always assigned to nursing homes they or their caregivers preferred. This was due to location, eligibility, affordability, or available space. Sometimes the only available venue was a nursing home listed as having serious problems. This listing was at sources such as the federal government's medicare.gov website. At nursing homes with problems, caregivers had to be particularly diligent regarding patients' care. At medicare.gov, information about quality measures, staffing, and state inspection results can be reviewed regarding specific nursing homes. Results of nursing home inspections are available at nursing homes and must be readily accessible.

ConsumerReports.org/nursinghomes is another source for evaluative nursing home information. Knowing information from various sources alerted caregivers to nursing home problems and helped them make informed decisions when choosing a nursing home. Caregivers also had to commit to involvement in planning care with the hospice team. Finally, they had to visit loved ones often.

Every patient needed at least one good advocate, someone to oversee healthcare. Patients who had the ability could be their own advocates at first, but when they could not handle the job themselves, others had to represent them responsibly. The primary caregiver was usually the authorized advocate.

Advocates had to be proactive in performing their duties, and they needed to keep good records. They had to gather information regarding the patient's condition and medications through personal research and inquiry. This information had to be shared with other relatives or friends who were caregivers, so everyone had basic information about the patient. Major decisions regarding patient care such as operations required informed choices. Monitoring the kinds of procedures involving patients was very important, particularly when medical personnel had to be reminded of patients' allergies and preferences.

The role of the caregiver can be a complicated potpourri of love, hatred, pride, guilt, joy, and resignation. Through the years, I've met many who served in that role for a variety of reasons:

1) "Mama did everything for us when we were growing up. She worked two jobs and went without, so we children could have a better life. My brother and I are honored to take care of her. He's with her as much as I am. We're just giving her the love and respect she gave us and everybody else. She raised us to do good for others. Doing good for her now when she needs us is our blessing, too."

2) "If you look at who's taking care of my daddy now, you wouldn't know he had three other children besides me. The others hardly do anything for him, and I'm always asking them to help out. Before you start thinking he was a bad father when we were growing up, let me tell you he wasn't. If you want to know the truth, he was too good to us. My trifling sisters and brothers just took him for granted. Now, they know Daddy is confused with Alzheimer's disease, so they use that as another excuse not to come see him. They figure he won't miss them. My siblings are a disgrace. Everything is on me."

3) "My mother was the kind of person who never should have had children. She was into drugs and the fast life for as long as I can remember. As a child, I prayed for her to change, but she never did. She left us alone a lot, even at night. Finally, my grandmother stepped up and raised us. Bless her soul, she died six years ago. We made sure she didn't want for anything. Now, my mother's dying, and I'm the only one who will come see about her. My sisters and brothers say she's getting what she deserves for all those

years she chose dope over us. I don't judge them, because I know how they feel. I'm still angry with her myself, but I come see about her anyway. I guess I want to be a better person than she is."

4) "We held a family meeting when Mom and Pops continued to deteriorate healthwise. They had reached the stage where they couldn't live alone any longer. Mom almost burned the house down, and Pops started roaming all over the neighborhood asking people where he lived. At the meeting, everybody had reasons why they couldn't be primary caregivers. They either lived out of town or had other obligations they said interfered. Several of them mentioned that I lived in town and didn't have as many responsibilities as they did. I don't know how they could make assumptions like that about what's going on in my life. I don't tell them most of my personal business. Anyway, I finally agreed to be the primary caregiver, but only if they would all make a written commitment with me. We made a list of what everybody would do to help on a regular basis. I can truthfully say they all are doing what they promised, including contributing money to our parents' care. Knowing I can always count on them helps me a lot. If they could fully understand, my parents would be proud of the way we are handling things."

Most people didn't set out to become caregivers. Some enjoyed nurturing their patients and found the caregiving experience challenging, but rewarding. Others were depressed and felt trapped in a hole with no way out, except the death of persons in their care. Negative feelings led to guilt that compounded their problems. Caregivers received their roles in various ways. Some were assigned because of their rank or gender in the family. Family members tended to put pressure on older siblings or females in the family to be designated caregivers. Living in a geographical location in proximity to patients' nursing homes was another factor that narrowed the caregiver selection to particular people. Finally, there were situations where there was no one else available or no one else available who would take the responsibility for being a caregiver. Some caregivers were paid guardians with no family ties to patients who were assigned to them legally. While some paid guardians were dedicated, others had little commitment to advocate for or even visit their patients regularly.

How caregivers received their assignments and accepted them was often a determining factor in how content they would be in adjusting to the inevitable difficulties that arose. Caregiving required a commitment to learning new skills, controlling ongoing frustration, and unselfish giving to continually declining patients. Efforts were seldom balanced with appreciation from others, particularly from those patients who had dementia. If caregivers did not receive help for their excessive negative feelings, they could take their anger out on others, including patients. They could also find themselves physically unhealthy and emotionally distraught. Some caregivers felt lonelier than patients and overwhelmed with their duties.

The good health of patients is connected to the good health of caregivers. Stress increases susceptibility to strokes and heart disease. Caregivers have to be flexible and willing to ask for assistance when they need it. They have to accept that other people don't do things the way they do them. Many caregivers work full or part-time jobs and need help themselves. Some eventually have to apply at their jobs for family and medical leaves that entitle them to a limited number of weeks per year of unpaid leave for family caregiving without losing their job security or health benefits. Other caregivers are able to use flextime at their jobs, change shifts with coworkers, or do job-sharing.

On a regular basis, caregivers need to evaluate how they are doing in terms of sleep, irritability, tiredness, isolation, depression and tolerance levels. They should be conscious of taking care of themselves by balancing their lives. The hospice team is available to help caregivers with suggestions and supportive referrals such as counseling and support groups.

The duties of caregiving can be divided among several people. Those who can help may be more willing if they are approached and offered a specific assignment after discussion about their preferences. Some may prefer to help during a particular time of day and only perform certain kinds of tasks that they do well. A little accommodation can go a long way in making caregiving a win-win situation for everybody involved.

Those who cannot visit regularly can find other ways to contribute to the caregiving process. They can make phone calls, give financial assistance, babysit, cook, do errands, and perform other work that assists those who visit the nursing home frequently. Caregiving is so complex that there is some aspect in which everyone can participate after they decide to become involved. Having a major role in improving the quality of someone else's life can be very satisfying.

I noticed that most caregivers visited during the day or right after work. They usually had to leave early at night to get home to their families. I advised caregivers to visit patients at daytime and nighttime whenever they could. By going at night, they would become acquainted with a different shift of workers whom they would never meet during the day. These workers tended to have fewer patient advocates to critique what they did. I thought that having caregivers visit both day and night at unscheduled times improved patient advocacy. By covering various times, caregivers could increase their ability to monitor patients' conditions and treatment more effectively.

Some caregivers and patients assume that doctors and nurses know everything there is to know about treatment of a particular illness. This myth is sometimes perpetuated by society. When lives are literally given over to the care of others with no questions asked, the stage is set for potential success or catastrophe, depending on the skills of the professionals in charge. Doctors and nurses are people first. They have their own beliefs about life, death, and pain management that may or may not coincide with the hospice philosophy. They come with a range of physical and mental abilities. Some may be very skilled and caring. Others may be much less skilled or uncaring for a variety of reasons. Sometimes appearances can be deceptive.

Having an awareness of some of the problems previously mentioned regarding the healthcare system should be reason enough for every caregiver to personally become familiar with information and procedures involving patients. One way to do this is to ask questions that provide more specific details in the answers. If a particular procedure is to be done that causes concern, the medical professional should be asked why it should be done, what the expected outcomes are for the patient, and what the potential side effects are. A notebook should be used to record important information. Caregivers can do their own follow-up research on the Internet, at the library, or through other medical consultation.

Patients often have problems that need attention from nurse aides, caregivers, or volunteers, depending on the nature of the problem. Unusual or serious concerns should always be reported to nursing home and hospice professionals. These are a few common areas I noticed and how they should be addressed:

- Appearance: Patients' overall appearance should be evaluated regularly. They should be clean, have their hair combed and skin moisturized when dry. Clothes should be appropriate and neat.

- Nail Care: Patients should have nails, including toenails, cleaned and trimmed as needed. Neglect in this area should be reported.

- Dry Mouth: Not only can dry mouth be uncomfortable, it can cause infection if neglected. Moistening a washcloth to clean the lips and rinsing the mouth with water can be very helpful in raising the level of patients' comfort. Patients who are able should be encouraged to drink liquids, especially during hot weather.

- Complaints: Patients' symptoms such as pain, constipation, diarrhea, itching, and nausea should be reported, so the causes of their concerns can be investigated.

- Boredom: Patients should have activities available to them that keep them engaged in life and help their self-esteem as much as possible. Even bedridden patients can be exposed to activities of interest. While patients are alive, the quality of their life is of utmost importance.

I met many family members at nursing homes. Most were relatives of patients other than the person I was visiting. These were often people who came several times a week to visit a few hours. Most were very devoted to their ill relatives. They brought homecooked meals, clean clothes, and very protective attitudes when it came to how their loved ones were treated. Frequent visits reassured patients of their importance as family members.

Caregivers of patients with forms of dementia had additional concerns. A major problem was getting hospice care for them. Determining patients' future life spans was difficult, and the predicted life span for hospice patients is six months. Family and friends of patients with dementia often had a hard time accepting their loved ones' condition. It was disconcerting not being recognized by people who had known them all their lives. Adult children found it painful to be around parents who treated them like strangers and asked, "Who are you? Why are you in my room? Do your know where my children are?" These questions were like knives in their hearts. Not getting positive emotional feedback from patients made some caregivers feel more stressed.

Some relatives and friends of patients used dementia as an excuse to decrease or end visits. They justified their absence by saying patients wouldn't realize they hadn't visited or that they didn't want to see loved ones they had known so many years "in that condition." They had difficulty accepting the reality that their loved ones were ill and needed the same compassion they would be given if they had any other illness. Dementia can sometimes be harder on family and friends than on patients.

Instead of focusing on what patients have lost, loved ones should focus on what patients still have left. They need to understand that their relationships with patients who have dementia must emphasize patients' needs. At the same time, they have to be aware of their own needs for balance in their lives and accept supports that are available. Sometimes caregivers die before patients do. Adult daycare is one option for creating respite relief time for both caregivers and patients.

In *Song of Solomon*, Nobel Laureate-winning author Toni Morrison writes, "What difference do it make if the thing you scared of is real or not?" I like this quote because it captures the essence of anybody's emotions, including those with dementia. Their experiences are as real as they see and feel them, and this must be acknowledged in responses to them. Patients reacted in a variety of ways to problems real or imaginary that they perceived. Some became hostile when threatened. Arguing with patients about what was real and what wasn't could be very exhausting for caregivers and upsetting to patients.

I found it was easier to humor patients, but that had to be done with caution. Depending on the degree of dementia that patients were experiencing at particular times, some were able to recognize when they weren't being told the truth and lost trust in that person. It was better to let patients come up with their own imaginary people and let them take the lead in developing their own fantasies. After they established the parameters, I joined in, depending on where I thought we might go in terms of safety.

Patients with dementia required a great deal of patience. They needed to be spoken to calmly without pressure, especially when they were frustrated. Sometimes when they became rebellious, it was the only way they knew how to express their frustration. It could have been a call for attention to a physical problem that needed to be addressed. It could have been a call for attention period. With staff shortages and so much staff turnover, patients often wanted to be noticed in a special way. Patients with dementia were usually aware of their surroundings on some level. That's why their behavior couldn't be viewed simply as combative without further analysis.

Maintaining the self-esteem of persons with dementia is important. They need a strong sense of being loved and accepted unconditionally, even when they are not understood, within the limitations of their behavior. A regular daily routine, in which they are encouraged to use their capabilities and experience pleasure, works best for them. They like schedules and rituals. One patient always wanted her blanket tucked in and pulled up to her neck before I left. Another had a specific route she wanted to take on her wheelchair rides. Patients with dementia need stimulation and interesting things to do, just like other people. Simple creative activities related to events, the arts, and places from their personal backgrounds seem most attractive to them. People and experiences that remind them of the past help them to connect with who they are as people.

A famous American actress named Lena Horne said, "It's not the load that breaks you down, it's the way you carry it." Attitude is everything. Two people can experience exactly the same circumstances and respond in totally different ways. One reason for that is the uniqueness of each person's experience. Attitude impacts responses. People have to consciously remind themselves that they can choose how they will respond to difficult situations. This is not always easy, especially on a daily basis or during the middle of a crisis. But they can get better over time. Patients with dementia can be very challenging. It helps when caregivers pause and consciously choose how they will carry the load.

I never took offense personally when patients with dementia were disagreeable with me. Patients became confused when they didn't understand what was happening to them or why something was happening around them. Their points of view always needed to be reviewed first to make sure their problems weren't caused by health issues they were unable to verbalize. Sometimes patients became bored and needed something creative to do.

When I was principal of an urban school with a high poverty level, people assumed it was probably very stressful making many decisions throughout the day. They were wrong. Making decisions was easy. I just asked myself, "What's in the best interest of students?" and the right answer always showed up. Caregivers can do the same thing. They should gather as much information as they can, so all their decisions about patients will be informed ones. Then they should ask themselves the most important question: "What's in the best interest of the person in my care?" The answer will wave at them.

Relatives and friends work best together when they all understand and accept individual contributions everyone makes for the good of patients. They cooperate more when they keep communication lines open and don't make assumptions about others' intentions. Holding meetings with agendas and ground rules regarding interruptions and other courtesies is helpful. If communication begins to break down, caregivers should voice their concerns, trying not to argue or ignite family dysfunctions.

Caregivers need support from family, friends, and anyone else who may be concerned and want to help. These people can make phone calls, take caregivers out for enjoyment, offer financial assistance, stay with patients, bring meals, and run errands. Most of all, everyone involved, whether caregivers or supporters, should make patients' quality of life their priority.

Deeper Than Words

The outside world arrives
wearing my willing face.
Toothless, your smile widens
like a baby's hungry for attention.
Almost ninety-eight years old,
your inner candle still glows.

A hospice volunteer, I lean closer,
talk into your listening left ear,
"Today is Sunday, Miss Loretta."
My news drifts away like smoke.
You stare at me through dying coals.
Whatever I ask, you whisper, "Yes."

I stroke your age-softened arms
while your hazed mind masters sleep.
Watching you, I dream generations
of women black and strong, each one
a book of sustaining stories
about joy, pain, courage, survival.

Within your warm brown frame,
spirits from our common history linger.
Aides say you have dementia,
that you don't know a word I say.
Our language goes deeper than words.
We speak to each other's souls.

—Frances Shani Parker

11	# Death # Journey	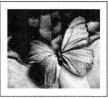

"Mama, you and Daddy are senior citizens, and I've been thinking about what should be done if something happened to one or both of you. Suppose you were dying, what kind of medical treatment would you want? What about your funeral, burial, and your possessions? How can your wishes be carried out if nobody knows them?"

"I always said you worry too much. Your daddy and I have our health challenges, just like everybody else. There is plenty of time in the future for that kind of talk. I don't even want to think about any of us passing, and you shouldn't either. It's too depressing. And don't go bringing it up to your daddy, getting him all upset."

Attempts to talk about death are met with resistance too often. But death is inevitable, and it is wise to be prepared. Ideally, preparations for death should be made long before illness even comes. Patients and caregivers should discuss plans for death and make necessary arrangements. Medical advances that extend lives artificially are readily available, so caregivers should arrange to address end-of-life care wisely. This is not always easy to do. After years of avoidance, some patients refuse to rise from their beds of denial. Caregivers must think of creative ways to approach the subject of death preparations. To continue to ignore the discussion will only make matters harder later on. Healthcare professionals can assist those who need help.

Written advance directives are important legal documents that should be completed. These documents can be done long before a patient is ill:

- The *healthcare power of attorney*, also known as the durable power of attorney for healthcare, is the document that designates the healthcare proxy, who is the person assigned to make medical decisions for the patient when the patient is no longer able to do

so. A patient should get this person's permission before assigning this responsibility. No one can be
forced to be a healthcare proxy. This person should
not be a member of the patient's healthcare team.

- The *living will*, states the patient's wishes regarding
  the administration of end-of-life medical treatment
  when the patient is not able to do so.

- A written *healthcare advance directive* combines the
  healthcare power of attorney, the living will and
  other information, including instructions for organ
  and tissue donations.

Advance directives are important in guiding medical
professionals in how to treat patients in such situations as
resuscitation. While some patients may want aggressive
medical treatment, others may not. Patients can modify
these directives at any time. Healthcare providers are legally responsible for honoring advance directives, and they
should be held accountable for implementing them. However, there is no guarantee that procedures patients requested will always be followed. That's why caregivers
must be vigilant in keeping abreast of procedures involving
patients and making patients' written requests available.

Caregivers can contact local medical facilities for information on the appropriate documents for advance directives. They are not the same in every state. Forms can also
be obtained from state health departments, legal offices,
and on the Internet. Most states require that the documents be witnessed. An attorney, while not required, can
also prepare documents in preparation for death.

Medical advance directives are not connected with patients' property. When patients die, there must be some
way to determine who gets property they leave behind.
Probate is the process that proves the existence of a valid
will or determines who legal heirs are otherwise. A will is a
legal document that explains how to distribute property
after death. The executor named in a will is the person
designated to be in charge of handling personal affairs of

the deceased. A well prepared will, often done by an attorney, makes legal procedures faster and easier after a patient dies. When no will is left, state law determines how assets and property will be distributed. Probate court handles this process. It can take months and involves attorney and court costs. A formal will can decrease time and costs. Certain types of property allocated to specific beneficiaries do not go through probate or, if they do, the process is much more simplified.

Another kind of will that more people are considering is an ethical will. This will, which can be written or tape recorded informally, includes values, morals, and wishes that someone bequeaths or hands down to others. While it is not legally binding, an ethical will provides a wonderful opportunity to pass on a legacy from one generation to the next, across generations, and beyond family members. Conveying this information, which may include stories, can be very comforting, particularly for a hospice patient. It's a personal way of letting relatives and friends know one's ethical intentions that are not connected to material inheritance. For example, a father might encourage his children to be good parents or will them the courage to make just decisions in life. Relatives might be asked to continue positive family traditions. Family members and friends might be advised to improve by incorporating more positive behaviors that have been lacking.

Having patients' wishes in writing allows caregivers to understand and implement exactly what patients want. Copies of important documents should be given to those who will need them, and copies should be kept in locations where they can be found readily when needed. Papers are put away and not available at critical times too often.

Some patients want to play an active role in planning their own funerals or memorial services, including selecting clothes they will wear, choosing the roles of participants, and writing their own obituaries. They can also be involved in planning activities related to cemeteries, caskets, and urns after cremations. Patients may be interested in donating their bodies or organs. Most medical schools need donations of whole bodies for research and instruction. Organs can be donated to keep other people alive. Patients' input should be encouraged because it helps them bring closure to dying and reassures them of getting the kind of treatment and services they want. It also comforts them to know they are not leaving others to do these tasks after they die.

Diann, one of my hospice patients, was a good example of this. She was all ready to go to heaven, but she kept putting off dying because she wanted her death ritual and related plans to be in order.

"I won't be here when you come next week. I'll be in heaven. You can call ahead if you want to be sure I'm not here. That way you won't make a trip here for nothing," Diann warned me. "Thanks for telling me. I'll just come anyway and see for myself," I responded like being warned about someone's upcoming death was common. Lately, every time I left from visiting her, she said it was the last time I would see her, because she would be dead before I returned the following week.

When I returned and she was still alive, I'd say, "Well, I guess you changed your mind about dying this week." Diann always had a good excuse. Sometimes she hadn't died because she didn't want to miss a festive activity such as the annual Christmas party. But most times, it was for practical reasons like getting her funeral, burial, and other after-death plans in order. She wanted her children to clean her house thoroughly, so relatives and friends could go there to fellowship after her funeral. Cleaning entailed sorting and packing clothes for charity. Then there was the selection of a casket, songs, speakers, her dress, etc. My weekly warnings continued for months.

Diann even invited me to join her on her death journey, saying it might be more fun if we went together. I passed on this, saying it just wasn't my time. I reminded her that she already had plenty of people there waiting for her. In case I had any other ideas, she reminded me that she couldn't hold a place for me there because I'd have to earn one myself.

One day, her warning came true. I received the hospice phone call saying she had died. All I could do was laugh to myself and say, "Good for you, Diann! You finally did it!

Sometimes relatives and friends don't know how to respond to dying patients. They are uncomfortable, nervous about saying the wrong thing, condescending toward them, maybe even afraid to be around them. I have noticed that frequently patients are ignored while caregivers and others discuss them in their presence. Even when patients are visibly awake and capable of speaking for themselves, caregivers often answer questions for them. The following recommendations can serve as a guide for treatment of the dying:

- People should be mindful of the fact that dying people often sense how others feel. While patients may make every effort to help them feel relaxed and not burdened by their illnesses, dying people have enough to do just dealing with their own emotions and physical conditions relating to their illnesses. Therefore, family members and friends should treat dying loved ones in a normal fashion and with respect. Playing soothing music, reading, and talking to them, even when they do not respond, can be comforting to the dying at appropriate times. Hand massages with lotion can also be soothing.

- Caregivers should learn all they can about the illness, so they will be aware of symptoms and responses of patients. The more they know and understand about the illness and the resources of the healthcare community, the more comfortable they will be as caregivers. Levels of stress often increase when family members participate in decisions to withdraw support from the critically ill. Having accurate and realistic information regarding patients' conditions, particularly from the medical staff, prepares caregivers and others to be more receptive of outcomes, including death. It helps that hospice has many resources to assist patients and caregivers in preparation for end-of-life decisions.

- People around patients should never assume that those who are dying want them to make all of their decisions when they are capable of speaking for themselves. Most people want to be independent as long as possible.

- Caregivers should be patient and know that their efforts are appreciated, even when those who are dying may not always tell them. If dying people can respond to them, caregivers should ask for guidance or assurances that they are doing the right things.

- When it becomes necessary, caregivers should seek help from others who want to help, but who may not be clear about what they can do. Relatives and friends often welcome opportunities to help by doing specific tasks such as going on errands or relieving caregivers of bedside duties for awhile. Seeking help also includes taking advantage of resources through the healthcare community. Services and equipment are available through hospice to assist patients and their families.

- Family and friends should be aware that dying people want to be alone sometimes, so they can rest and process their own thoughts. On a personal level, death is a solo adventure that requires introspection and time for solitude.

The body knows when it's time to slow down and die. Each body will die in its own way and in its own time when the process starts. Among symptoms of impending death, there might be decreases in food intake, swallowing, communication; and increases in sleep, weakness, and spiritual awareness. The latter might include speaking to, looking at, or dreaming about persons who have already died. Patients may become incontinent, agitated, confused, withdrawn, and congested. Bright light in patients' eyes should be avoided. Patients should be turned gently when necessary.

All people are entitled to a comfortable, pain-free death. This includes patients who can verbalize how they feel and those who can't. Pain is only one of several symptoms that patients may be experiencing. Shortness of breath, delirium, and fatigue from weight loss are a few others. Emotionally, severe pain can cause patients to experience anger, frustration, fear, anxiety, and depression. Hospice care should provide every reasonable effort to control pain and stabilize patients to a plateau of comfort.

The hospice nurse or doctor can explain any changes that cause concern during the dying process. Some caregivers become upset when dying patients lose their appetites. Because they view food as nurturing, they want to keep giving patients more food than they need. It is important to keep in mind that dying patients with little or no appetite are not starving or in pain from hunger in the manner that is commonly understood. They are responding normally to the body's breaking down as part of the dying process. Swallowing may be difficult for them and could lead to choking when food is forced into their mouths. They could also become nauseous and vomit from being forced to take in food they do not want. Dying patients may also want less to drink. The insides of their mouths can be moistened with droplets or a fine spray, and a lip cream can be used, especially if they are breathing through their mouths. It is not unusual for breathing of dying patients to fluctuate from quiet to noisy or to have an irregular rhythm.

As much as possible, caregivers should remain calm and give patients reassuring presence. Although patients may not want to talk themselves, they may appreciate supportive talking by others explaining who is in the room, how they feel, what is going on around them. Too much company from those not close to dying patients, however, could be tiring.

Families and friends sometimes make the mistake of thinking that patients who appear to be asleep or in a coma cannot hear or comprehend what those present are saying in the room. Hearing is one of the last senses to leave. Conversations around sleeping or dying patients should always be monitored because there is a possibility that patients will hear what is being said. Many patients are consoled knowing that their loved ones support their decision to let go and die. Some find prayers or music comforting during this time.

One activity that may need to be scheduled is emergency air travel for those who might want to visit the terminally ill person before death. This can also be done after the patient dies to assist travelers in getting to the location of the death ritual. Some airlines have bereavement or compassion fares available for family members traveling for an imminent or actual death. These fares are discounted off the full price, but may not be the lowest fares available. Information regarding the ill or deceased person, the traveler's relationship with that person, the physician, healthcare institution, and funeral home might be requested.

Numerous tasks must be done after death, and they should be done thoughtfully in an unrushed manner. If possible, the exact time of death should be recorded. Some may want to spend time with the deceased. Nursing homes will have procedures to follow regarding death. Family members, hospice staff, and possibly others such as a spiritual advisor and a mortuary for funeral arrangements should be notified. Several certified copies of death certificates will be needed to collect insurance and other death benefits. These copies can be obtained from mortuaries, vital statistics offices, county health departments, and online at county and state websites.

Family members may want to notify newspapers about publishing death notices and obituaries announcing the time and place of funeral or memorial services. Arrangements with an online memorial service, often affiliated with newspapers, can ensure that those who do not attend funeral or memorial services in person will have the opportunity to participate online. At a memorial website, guests can read the obituary, sign a guestbook, and view photographs. They can also send flowers, a sympathy gift, or a charity donation in the deceased person's name. A record, including the names and information of those who send condolences, flowers, etc., should be kept for later thank-you notes.

Contact should be made with insurance companies, unions, fraternal organizations, government offices, banks, credit unions, and real estate agencies to change titles if necessary. Employee benefits from all previous employers should be investigated.

Arrangements for child care and out-of-town guests must be considered. Food may be another consideration. In many families, relatives, friends, and church members often assist in providing food after funerals.

In the midst of all this activity, family members and friends must also consider their own feelings about death and the person who has died. The occasion that they have been expecting while the loved one was ill has finally come. A life has been lived. A sun has set. Someone has come face to face with the Other Side of Through.

Invisible Train

People live and die,
leave parts of themselves
hidden in our souls. They travel
like trains to inner stations,
remain in memory depots forever.

I remember when we coupled,
anticipated a journey
with unending scenic routes.
Turbulent disagreements
sidetracked love's destination.
Foul weather of illness
delayed steady movement.

Your body lies buried,
but your absence is an illusion.
You will always be an invisible train
that my soul will remember
with bitter sweetness.

—Frances Shani Parker

12	Death Rituals	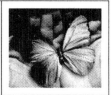

Death rituals have always been woven into the fabric of America. While different cultures have responded in numerous ways, the need to honor the deceased in an atmosphere of healing and support from others has been a common manner for mourning the dead. A powerful message sent to mourners during death rituals is the physical mortality of life.

Many years ago, death rituals in America were a continuation of the family's natural involvement with the deceased at home. Families were caregivers to their ill loved ones. They saw caregiving as their responsibility to family members. Home was considered the best place to die.

After a death took place, the body of the deceased was prepared at home for viewing in the living room. Mourners came to pay their respects, console the family, and offer other forms of assistance. The family appreciated this outpouring of support from the community. After the funeral, the body was buried in the family cemetery or in a natural setting. No undertakers were needed to handle death rituals. It never dawned on relatives that they couldn't handle everything well themselves. They had been successful at performing these services many years.

Involvement with death-ritual arrangements was and still is therapeutic, but rituals are handled in a different manner. Fewer people die at home. It is common for them to die in institutions such as hospitals and nursing homes. They die with or without relatives or friends present. The immediate future after death often includes a death ritual, such as a funeral or memorial service that recognizes, honors, and brings closure to a loved one's death.

Family members usually have little desire or confidence in their own abilities to orchestrate a wake, funeral, and burial themselves. Reluctant to handle death arrangements, they prefer to pay an undertaker, also referred to as a funeral director, for that service. Undertakers retrieve the body and work with the family in planning death rituals. The average funeral costs several thousand dollars. This doesn't include other related expenses such as a burial plot and headstone. Even though most states do not require that an undertaker be involved when someone dies, some family members feel compelled by tradition to hire an undertaker.

People should be very careful when making funeral and burial decisions, particularly during the vulnerable periods right before and after a loved one has died. Emotions might be flooded with guilt or a burning desire to please the deceased. This could cloud the reality of what really needs to be purchased at reasonable prices. Detailed explanations should be given during transactions. With options to purchase such services as touch-screen videotaped biographies of the deceased for permanent cemetery viewing, there could be a tendency to overspend. Medallions with digitally stored biographical information and pictures can be made available for others to download data at the gravesite. Information about the deceased can be displayed for mourners to read on their hand-held computers. With prices of burials and cremations steadily increasing, it is little wonder that funeral arrangements and burials generate billions of dollars annually.

A security precaution related to death rituals includes the possibility of crimes being committed while rituals are being held and mourners are away from their homes. Unfortunately, we live at a time when some people wait for opportunities such as funerals or memorial services to burglarize homes when all occupants will be gone. Even when death announcements are not published in newspapers, information regarding the times and places of death rituals often becomes widespread. It's a good idea to have someone available to keep watch at home when family members are gone.

Funerals and memorial services are occasions for relatives and friends to eulogize, sing, pray, read sacred texts, or share anecdotes about the deceased. Although they may have religious connections, death rituals do not need religious components. Atheists, people who do not believe in the existence of gods, perform death procedures in ways that reflect their beliefs. Many atheists prefer to have their bodies cremated or donated to science.

Rituals inspired by religion usually have a member of the clergy officiate. Flowers and plants sent by relatives and friends are often displayed. Some families request that a financial donation be made to a charity in lieu of donating flowers. The life of the deceased is usually praised, and the family is offered comfort. The officiating clergy may also use this time to remind mourners about their own need to get their spiritual houses in order. Families can create rituals that meet their needs when the wishes of the deceased are unknown.

People sometimes attach fear to certain rituals and practices connected with death. For example, cemeteries and corpses continue to be viewed as sources of gloom and terror. These learned experiences become incorporated into thoughts at an early age and are not natural to the death experience itself. Children should be taught positive information regarding death, so they will have healthy perspectives about the life and death process. When appropriate for them, children should be present at death rituals. They need to have their grief addressed and they can benefit from this growth opportunity.

Many Christians in African American communities refer to funerals as "homegoing" services because the deceased is going home, crossing over to the other side, making a transition to the spirit world. Emotions may run high at funerals as mourners are moved by the music and spiritual energy, which builds up as the service progresses. Various family members and friends eulogize the deceased. Although there is sadness because the loved one is no longer physically available, there is joy in knowing that the deceased has gone to a better place where there will be no more sorrow and where everyone will be reunited one day.

Many people believe that they can still communicate on some level with the loved one who died, and are consoled by this knowledge. Funerals are often followed by burial services at cemeteries. Later, mourners meet at the home of a family member or another fellowship location to reminisce and share refreshments and stories about the deceased. Humorous stories often add a joyous perspective as attempts are made to build a bridge over the valley of death.

The popularity of jazz funerals in New Orleans has enhanced this city's reputation for uniqueness. Usually held for musicians, members of social and pleasure clubs, and community leaders, jazz funerals are occasions for the larger community to join with relatives and friends in honoring the deceased. Mourners come prepared to render a dynamic farewell commemoration, which might last for several days. Death is an event that requires rejoicing, and a jazz funeral in New Orleans epitomizes that sentiment.

After services at the church or funeral home, a grand marshal leads a brass band and an assembled group of mourners, along with the hearse, in a procession to the cemetery to "drop the body." The band plays solemn music such as "Just a Closer Walk with Thee." Stepping unhurriedly with the beat, participants walk a route down city streets. If the cemetery is far away, they only walk several blocks. When they reach the cemetery, they "cut the body loose" as the hearse slowly enters for final services where the body is laid to rest.

Later, after the procession of mourners leaves the cemetery, a rousing celebration begins with the band playing an upbeat song like "When the Saints Go Marching In." The funeral procession continues, growing in size with many community members, collectively called "second liners," who join in the joy with curious bystanders. A spirited dance called the "second line" is prominent among the celebrants. Various bars are visited as they continue their festivities through the streets. Many participants bob umbrellas, some brightly decorated, and wave handkerchiefs in the air to the hot-sauce beat of the music. Surely, the deceased must be ecstatic with the large turnout of well-wishers expressing such jubilance in the send-off.

Death rituals are performed in a variety of ways among various cultures and religions. Differences often exist within racial, ethnic, and religious groups because ultimately people are individuals influenced by their families, age, religion, economic status, and geographic locations. For example, there are different denominations of Judaism. These differences impact how individual Jews view medical treatment, death, and death rituals.

Jewish families bury their dead as quickly as possible. Embalmment and cremation are not allowed. They may want to perform certain rituals, such as washing the body during or after the time of death. The body may not be left alone from the time of death until after the burial. The brief funeral includes recitation of memorial prayers and a eulogy. The public may not view the body. A period of mourning follows.

Muslims wash the body of the deceased during a special purification ritual. My friend Carolyn, who is not a Muslim, participated in the washing of her Muslim husband's body and received great comfort through her involvement. I asked her about her participation in this moving death ritual.

She explained, "The Imam, a Muslim leader, mentioned that three adults, including a spouse, could wash the body of the deceased during a ritual that prepares the loved one for being with Allah. He asked if I wanted to go to the funeral home and be a participant in washing Melvin, my deceased husband. I welcomed this opportunity. I knew Melvin would have wanted me to be actively involved. In a private room at the funeral home, I used soap and water to clean Melvin's upper body, while the Imam and another gentleman washed his lower body. During the washing process, I spoke tenderly to Melvin. I told him how wonderful he looked and how much I loved him. Even though he was dead, he wore the most beautiful smile. I knew he heard every word I said. The room was very quiet and serene. After three complete body washings, Melvin's body was dried, oiled, and wrapped in two pieces of white cloth. A final covering displayed writings of the Holy Quran."

"How did you feel about your role during this ritual and afterward?" I inquired.

"What I felt most while washing Melvin was an inner sense of calm. I knew his wishes were being carried out, not only with that ritual, but with all the Muslim rituals related to his death. As I washed him, I knew he was at peace. I remembered how bad his pain had been sometimes before he died. He had prayed aloud to Allah to have mercy on him during his suffering. I felt relief knowing his distress was over. I appreciated the respect he was given. Washing Melvin's body was a blessing that helped me in my healing."

While so-called traditional American funerals still exist, our changing society continues to reflect people's preferences to personalize death rituals in ways that differ from the norm. More and more Americans who perceive themselves as spiritual, but not religious, are adapting their death rituals accordingly. With increasing activities being held at funeral homes, changes have been made in the order and location of services. Other innovations include more contemporary music and the use of more technology such as videos. Although burials are both above and below ground in cemeteries, the dead are being disposed of in a wide range of ways.

Growing up in New Orleans, I thought cemeteries everywhere had people buried above the ground. Some people said that a long time ago, the city tried to bury more people below the ground, just like most cities do. But due to the city's high water level, the caskets would rise up from the graves on dark rainy nights. Residents said it was eerie seeing caskets floating through the streets like haunted boats. Like many stories I heard during childhood, I wasn't sure if this was another story drenched in New Orleans folklore.

One of my hospice patients told me an interesting cemetery story that she related with great sincerity. Joan had several unusual qualities about her that made me wonder. At sixty-five, she was the youngest patient assigned to me after years of hospice volunteering. Her name was the same as my grandmother's, and I had her grandmother's name. When we made these discoveries during our first meeting, we took them as signs that we were destined to have a great patient and volunteer relationship. In time, I learned that the most unusual thing about Joan was what she said.

"Is your mother alive?" Joan asked me one day.

"No, she died a few years ago in her eighties," I replied.

"You know, you can still be with her and talk to her if you want to."

"Oh, I know we can still communicate."

"No, I mean for real. You can be with her in person. Just get her clothes together and her shoes. Don't forget her coat. They say it's cold outside. Take them to the cemetery where she's buried. Just set them on top of her grave and wait. She'll rise out of her grave and put them on. Then you can take her home with you. In every way, she'll look just like the real person you knew. Other people won't be able to see her, but you will."

"Hmmm. I've never heard that before."

"Most people haven't. I know about it because I did it with my two grown sons. They were both murdered in a drive-by shooting on the same day. I didn't know how I would get through the pain. Finally, I took their clothes to the cemetery and did what I just told you. Both of them went home with me. It was the best day of my life. I got my sons back." Satisfied, she smiled.

Some people will dismiss this story as crazed comments of a demented woman. But if you really listen, you'll hear the impressive empowerment in her words.

Instead of being buried at a cemetery, increasing numbers of people are choosing cremations, in which bodies are reduced to bone fragments as a result of intense heat and flames. Sometimes families are allowed to be present at cremations. Not only are cremations selected because they are less expensive than traditional burials, some prefer them for the ease in spreading the ashes and the convenience in incorporating cremated remains into death rituals. Most religions accept cremations and permit the cremated remains or cremains, as they are called, at memorial services. Cremains can also be buried in a cemetery plot, stored in a mausoleum, or scattered somewhere such as a garden or a body of water. They are often stored by families who keep them in holders that vary in uniqueness. These may include such containers as vases with pedestals or personalized teddy bears with hidden pouches for ashes. Ashes of loved ones are also being used in jewelry, shotgun shells, and fireworks.

A growing number of alternative-death businesses advocate home funerals and burials in natural environments referred to as "green cemeteries" that promote decomposition. Some people have lost confidence in managing death arrangements themselves, but they still want to exercise this option by learning how to correctly perform procedures after death. They attend presentations held by businesses that teach them how to properly prepare a dead body. All techniques are natural, including no embalming of the body. Another alternative-death business advocates cryonics, a procedure in which dead bodies are frozen. This is done with hopes that medical advances in the future will cure illnesses and extend lives of those deceased.

According to the U.S. Department of Veterans Affairs, members who die while on active duty, veterans honorably discharged, reservists, and National Guard members may be eligible for burial in a U.S. Department of Veterans Affairs national cemetery. Spouses and minor children of service members and veterans may also be eligible for burial in a national cemetery. Reservations in advance for gravesites are not allowed. Cemeteries for veterans are operated by many states. Veterans Affairs will furnish free headstones and markers worldwide for graves of eligible veterans or service members who die on active duty and, in certain cases, provide them for their spouses and dependents.

Impromptu memorials, which have been around for many generations in this country, are increasing. Publicized terrorists' attacks, natural disasters, crimes, and accidents have united large numbers of people around common bonds of grief. These memorials often begin with a tragedy involving one or more deaths. For example, a child might be murdered or killed in a car accident. Within a short period of time, toys such as stuffed animals, along with flowers, balloons, posters, cards, photographs, and other memorial displays begin to accumulate at the site where the crime or accident took place. At some point, community members may come together at that same location or elsewhere for a candlelight vigil of prayers for the deceased as well as prayers for community healing and improvement. The shrines and altars resulting from impromptu memorials touch many people in a personal manner and serve as powerful reminders of the deceased and the cause represented.

An aura of heartache blanketed the air at the September 11, 2001 wall of memorials in New York City. At the site where the World Trade Center twin towers stood before they became kindling targets for terrorists' fires, many sought healing by visiting the area and witnessing the memorial displays. I remember how extensive the displays were when I visited New York at the Ground Zero location a few months after the attack. Scattered images of casualties, thousands of love notes, and flowered tributes greeted visitors who came from all over the world. Among the clicking cameras were whispered memories spoken by those trying to bring closure to doors left ajar by trauma. These memorials served as multicultural expressions of grief. The following May after the tragedy, when recovery efforts ended for those who were killed but not found, a formal memorial procession and silent service were held. This solemn ritual, which included tolling bells, wailing bagpipes, and the playing of "Taps," was televised around the world.

Death rituals will continue to evolve with the passage of time. Choosing how to bring closure to the lives of deceased loved ones will become more personalized as increasing numbers of people are confronted with death-ritual decisions. People who die will be mourned and celebrated as relatives and friends unfasten their earthly connections with them.

Ground Zero

Scattered images of causalities,
thousands of love notes
blanket a former battlefield.
Whispered memories,
flowered tributes coax
closure of doors left ajar by trauma.

From my hotel window, I watch
the "Ground Zero" real-time movie
of a 21st century grave excavation
where the World Trade Center
rose and fell, a kindling target
for terrorists' fires.

Hills with human remains
transport like treasures
to a Staten Island landfill.
Conveying trucks beep
warning chants of danger
to a world in global doom denial.

I view the sixteen-acre hole
in the heart of a grieving nation,
listen to victims' voices
share their haunting horror:
"We fought to live and love,
trapped in a fatal inferno,
marooned in a tomb of ruins.
We nursed at the breast of fear
until our spirits were free."

—Frances Shani Parker

	Bereavement	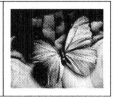
13	**Support**	

Although death is universal, people respond to it in countless ways. Even when they have been expecting someone's death for a long period of time, their reactions cannot be predicted. People grieve for different reasons. How they respond is closely connected with the kinds of relationships they shared with the deceased, their religious and cultural perceptions, how they cope with stress in general, and how the deceased died. Grieving might include varying degrees of emotional intensity that should be recognized as normal responses to death. Those left behind may also struggle with feelings of denial, guilt, anger, and depression.

Some family members and friends begin grieving before death actually comes. Depending on the circumstances, the illness may have served as a barrier that separated them from the deceased emotionally or physically over a period of time. Distancing themselves may have been how some caregivers coped with the ongoing stress caused by their responsibilities. By creating distance, they were able to lessen the full impact of pain. That separation may have been experienced as a kind of death.

In addition to the actual impending death, feelings of grief can be intermingled with fear about the future and how lives will be affected. Death could mean drastic lifestyle changes that appear overwhelming, particularly if there was a strong dependency on the deceased during day-to-day living. Through the years, many married couples have had only one spouse handle finances or make most decisions. In these situations, dependent spouses feel very vulnerable and afraid about their ability to manage and lead. If they have little or no experience working full-time, they could worry about how they will be able to make a living when their main source of income dies. This grieving before death may or may not impact the extent of grief that comes later.

Many people need little or no grief counseling, while others need extensive support for months or years. No timetable mandates when each person should start or finish. Some people stay in a state of denial for awhile and appear not to be grieving at all. While most people expect emotional grief displays, physical reactions such as fatigue, headaches, and tension may also be experienced. Because grieving can take such a physical and emotional toll, grievers should monitor how they are adjusting, keeping in mind that feelings should be faced, so healing can take place.

Occasionally, death is viewed as relief. Over a period of time, caregivers who have witnessed the deterioration and suffering of those in their care, along with their personal hardships relating to the illness, come to anticipate the sick person's peace and freedom. Knowing there is no medical cure for the continuing health decline, caregivers, particularly some who believe in a better afterlife, may begin to welcome death. It is not unusual to hear people say that they are glad a deceased loved one has finally found peace.

Children's grieving needs must be recognized and honored. Sometimes adults get so involved with handling personal emotions and situations arising as a result of the death that they lose awareness of what children might experience. Death can be overwhelming to children who are often limited in understanding death's finality and reasons. They may have difficulty expressing their confusion, fear, and sadness. Children need sensitive, age-appropriate and candid explanations about what has happened, along with comments about the future. Death should not be referred to as "going to sleep" because children might become anxious about sleeping. They need to be reassured that they are loved, that it is okay to be sad and share feelings with others. Most of all, they should know that their responses to death will be taken seriously.

For a period of time following death, relatives and friends may demonstrate generous support for those who are grieving. They might call or come by regularly to see how the bereaved are adjusting and help with children or out-of-town visitors. They may offer to write thank-you cards, go on errands, or bring meals for them. If it appears that some relatives and friends avoid contact with immediate family members of the deceased, they probably are avoiding them. Many people are so uncomfortable with death that they steer clear of conversations with those close to the deceased. Rather than approach someone who they know has had a loved one die recently, they might go down a different aisle in a store. Ordinarily, they could be talkative and social people, but if death becomes the topic, they struggle with what to say.

People who have difficulty in knowing what to do or say when communicating with those who have had loved ones die a short time ago need to realize that what matters most is that they demonstrate through words and actions that they care. The best things they can do are extend sympathy, offer to be available to help, and then let the grieving person guide the conversation. They should not impose their own religious views or decisions on what others should do in response to the death. Additional extended courtesies could include cards, invitations to go to a mutual place of enjoyment, and phone calls every now and then to see how the grieving person is doing. If the griever shows signs of depression or lack of adjustment progress, well-wishers can assist in getting help and support for them.

There comes a time when extensive support for grievers decreases as others move on with their own lives. This doesn't mean they no longer care, but it does speak to limitations on what others can give of themselves over time and still nurture and address their own needs as well as needs of those who depend on them. If grieving appears to be too much to handle without the extra ongoing attention supporters gave, it might be beneficial to get professional help, talk more with spiritual advisors, or join a support group. Grievers can also become involved in pleasurable activities, express feelings artistically, or talk with close friends and family members.

One important source of support for handling grief is the hospice team, particularly the chaplain and social worker. They are experienced in grief counseling and are familiar with the history of the deceased. Having bonded with patients and their caregivers, hospice team members often help by assisting families during the bereavement process. They know in general what to expect and how to respond. The hospice team wants to support patients and their families.

Some mourners suppress their own grief in an effort not to burden others. They may avoid talking about the deceased and convince themselves that, by ignoring the death, they will be able to move on faster with their lives. Grief needs to be recognized for what it is and dealt with accordingly. When it is suppressed, it will go undercover and resurface in another manner. Other aspects of lives also suffer when those who are grieving ignore them. Good health habits in eating, exercising, and leading a balanced life should be maintained at all times, but particularly during this period when grief can negatively impact health.

The holidays could be a troubling time for many grieving people, especially if they were involved in celebrating holiday traditions with the deceased. Through the years, people associate certain traditions with familiar faces and personalities. People and traditions become totally intertwined like a birthday cake with candles. They might go through the motions of celebrating, but internally may feel depressed because the deceased is no longer a part of the tradition. Deep down inside, they might want to avoid the whole holiday scene altogether. This is fine if they would be comfortable avoiding the holiday scene. But this option is not fine if it is only done as an escape from reminders about the deceased or because they are so miserable they don't know what else to do.

Mourners have to decide the best ways they can adjust to the holidays. One option is to create new holiday traditions. If holidays were celebrated as a family, new traditions can be planned as a family, so everyone can have input. This will give family members an opportunity to discuss their feelings about the deceased loved one and possibly include something in the new tradition that commemorates that person in an uplifting manner. This could be a type of memorial that adds pleasure to holidays in the future, something that would have pleased the deceased.

Whether celebrating the holidays alone, with others, or not at all, people should always follow their hearts and do what feels best for them. There is no one way for everyone. There are different ways that work well for different people. Some people who found the holidays stressful, phony, or too commercial before their loved one died may want to redirect their holiday focus. They might choose to participate in an activity that is calmer and more meaningful to them such as volunteering at places where they can help others or sharing with others in another capacity. Others may want to celebrate alone or with a few friends, take a trip to another state or country, or just be involved with something they enjoy doing that may or may not have anything to do with the holidays, but everything to do with their own quality of life.

Bereavement support has become quite extensive in the twenty-first century. Twenty years ago, most people probably never imagined that support would be available from unseen friends in cyberspace. More and more senior citizens are taking advantage of computer classes at senior centers and other locations. Relatives and friends are also helping them get connected to the cyber world of email, information surfing, shopping, and building websites.

Many bereavement support groups, message boards, and chat rooms are available on the Internet. While professional counselors operate at some websites, caution should always be exercised to determine which of the many sites are valuable. Memorial websites that honor deceased loved ones can be created or purchased for friends, family, and the general public to visit. Some memorial websites include virtual candles that can be lit to acknowledge anniversaries, birthdays, and other occasions. Before they die, the deceased loved ones can create e-mails and videos to be delivered periodically after death to cyberspace addresses. Numerous sites also exist for families and friends to share poetry, fiction, nonfiction, music, and photo albums related to the deceased.

Of course, traditional support that has withstood the passage of time is still available. For those who prefer this kind of assistance, support groups are available through hospice, medical facilities, churches, senior centers, and organizations such as the Alzheimer's Association. Other supportive resources include books, magazine articles, and newsletters available both online and at local stores.

Grieving family members and friends need time to sort out their feelings, make decisions about their own welfare, and plan for the future. This is not the time, however, to make major life-changing decisions unless they have been well planned beforehand. Death can cause some people to be vulnerable and make unstable choices. The bereaved should be careful not to become overly dependent on others or drugs, not to allow others to impose their beliefs on them, and not allow relatives or friends to make decisions for them that they can make for themselves.

While it is good to accept offers of help, primary attention should be on future adjustments with healthy independence. For some grievers, independence may include preparation for future employment, taking classes, or volunteering in order to feel more productive as a person. All decisions should be made carefully after considerable thought and research on the best choices to make.

Severe losses similar to death can be experienced through catastrophic acts of nature that also require bereavement support. On August 29, 2005, powerful Hurricane Katrina became the most destructive hurricane ever to strike in the United States. Garnering international attention, her massive fury devastated much of the Gulf Coast area in the South.

New Orleans, Louisiana's largest city, became a super bowl of toxic waters washing dreams away. Broken levees that had stood on guard for decades were no match for Katrina's strength, human incompetence, and speculated sabotage. Extensive flooding, accompanied by horrendous delays in governmental responses to assist and remove evacuees, submerged the city in disaster. Past pleas of "Throw me something, mister," commonly heard during the joyful Mardi Gras season, turned into desperate appeals of "Help us! Help us, please!" shouted by defenseless sufferers drowning in dread as they literally clung to life.

Few patients in nursing homes were evacuated before the levees broke. As flooding waters rose rapidly destroying homes, elderly and frail patients, many who were wheelchair-bound, bedridden, or dependent on generators for oxygen, were moved to higher floors in nursing homes where that option was available. Drinking water, food, medical supplies, and electricity became scarce as desperate hours evolved into nightmarish days with dead patients.

Many bodies were lost in the floods. Several months later, bodies continued to be discovered. Hundreds of thousands of residents were forced to leave what was left of their homes, if anything, and relocate elsewhere. Masses of evacuees were sent to cities where they knew no one and were totally dependent on the goodwill of strangers for their survival.

After the tragedy, residents who remained or returned to rebuild their city were confronted with the intensive care of collapsed or uninhabitable homes, many requiring continued mortgage payments. Houses wearing handwritten scrawls of body counts and frowning water lines expressed overwhelming misery. Receding waters left extreme mental pollution that further poisoned the city's health. Suicide rates and post-traumatic stress disorder

(PTSD) among adults and children escalated rapidly with few resources available for treatment. Piles of debris and abandoned cars waited in limbo, while Federal Emergency Management Agency (FEMA) trailers and blue plastic tarps on leaking roofs added to a surreal atmosphere.

Traumatized survivors experienced death, not only of their loved ones and lost material possessions, but also death of their communities, the city's unique vibe, and a way of life embedded in who they are. Those of us who live in other cities, but who cherish our New Orleans roots, also suffered a loss. While we were always aware of the city's many problems, we also remember happier times, life-changing harmonies with people, places, and events that swept us into sweetness, the way great New Orleans music does. The New Orleans we remember had died a brutal death.

Ultimately, grief is an individual matter that people must resolve at personal levels. They often require wound-healing time and a range of ongoing supports to worm their ways through mounds of immense loss to healthy recovery. Mourners should be patient with themselves and others, recognizing that, as they adjust to the death of a loved one or other loss, forward is still the direction in which they must move. The deceased would probably want them to do just that. Life is for living.

Love Poem from the Other Side of Through

Long before I died,
we walked together,
arms snaked around
each other's waists
like eels squeezing us
into oneness. We fed
each other words, marveled
at unquenchable passion
saturated with commitment.
Energized legs stepped
with harmony that misted
around us with each stride.
At the park, we relaxed
in a whirlpool of laughter.
Sunbeams disintegrated
steamy regrets. Waves of bliss
baptized born-again spirits,
filled us with the lovers' holy ghost.

—Frances Shani Parker

	Healthier Hospice	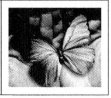
14		

It's time to use the "D" word, have open conversations about death. As science and technology discover more ways to extend human life, increasing numbers of people struggle with serious illnesses requiring hospice care. Future improvements of hospice are crucial for effectively meeting people's needs. Whether at home or in nursing homes, all people are entitled to benefits of excellent healthcare, particularly at critical times in their lives.

For many years, I have looked forward to the senior citizenship of baby boomers, people born from 1946-1964. I told myself it would be the first time in the history of this country that all elderly people would receive healthcare and other services they so richly deserve. The baby boomers are sneaking up on old age themselves, and elderly people tend to vote. Baby boomers are a powerful group in America. Collectively, they have the ability to light the lamp of justice for nursing home conditions and medical care of the elderly in general.

As caregivers of older relatives, many boomers are already acquainted with problems in the healthcare system. Unless corrective changes are made, boomers will be recipients of the same healthcare they complain about as caregivers. By that time, conditions will be worse because boomers will be coming in droves. Terminally ill patients and others in healthcare institutions need strong advocacy from boomers and all other segments of our society on a large scale. The increase in baby boomers creates an urgency to confront and solve healthcare problems, particularly those related to hospice and palliative care.

America is the only industrialized country that does not support a universal healthcare system. Millions walk around in constant fear of losing the coverage they have, of struggling with how to pay healthcare bills, and of worrying about how they will survive without healthcare. The latter group includes masses of people who have jobs that provide none. The elderly and ill suffer with their limited resources.

Hospice care must be expanded to include more palliative care for chronically ill patients. Treatment should include a natural evolution of health services for all patients who need them when they are terminally ill. People with incurable illnesses should not have to wait until a doctor officially determines in writing that they have six months to live. Too many patients are being referred very late during their illnesses or not at all.

The curative medical philosophy and the hospice philosophy are often like two men in love with the same woman. The curative man refuses to let her go, even though she has demonstrated her lack of commitment to him and her need to move on. The hospice man longs to stay with her because their relationship has reached a mutually meaningful level. The woman he loves embraces the fulfillment his hospice presence brings to her life. Some doctors and caregivers may be reluctant to admit that a patient cannot be saved. Patients may resist the prediction of their own death within months. Nursing home staff members who are focused on curing patients may not embrace the hospice philosophy of non-curative care.

In order to improve treatment of the terminally ill, nursing homes must commit to enhancing their expertise in certain hospice practices when they contract with hospice programs. This commitment must first come from the nursing home administrators. Services of the hospice team supplement those provided by the nursing home. Dying nursing home patients receive services more appropriate to their condition when they are in hospice care. In some cases, hospice practices naturally become part of the care given to terminal patients who are not assigned formally to a hospice program.

Funding for hospice programs is fundamental to their existence. They are businesses funded by the government or private insurance, grants from charitable organizations, and donations from the public and corporations. Not all insurance programs reimburse for hospice care and some only reimburse for particular services. Medicare, Medicaid, or private insurance financially reimburse hospice programs.

The majority of hospice services are reimbursed based on the number of days patients stay in the hospice program. When hospice patients are treated early, their initial costs are high and decrease as they stabilize. These higher initial costs must balance with lower stabilized costs over a period of months to maintain financial equity. When patients are continually referred late, accumulating high initial costs and dying shortly afterward without more days to stabilize at lower costs, financial imbalance results. Another financial concern is that non-profit charitable hospice programs are expected to care for patients who have no ability to pay. Obviously, changes must occur in how hospice programs are funded and when patients are referred.

Changing the concept of hospice among the general public will require widespread education on a national level. The business community could benefit economically by offering more support to hospice caregivers who want to continue to remain productive in the workforce, but have no options to consider. Many people have never heard of hospice or view hospice as a place to go when it's time to die. In order for more terminally ill and chronically ill patients to be treated for longer periods of time, hospice and palliative care must be viewed as advantageous services that provide compassion and comfort with broad medical outreach for diverse groups of people.

More doctors and related professionals must become comfortable with the hospice philosophy of providing quality care at the end of life when curative efforts are no longer viable. Medical schools are broadening training during residency and providing ongoing professional development to include far more information and hands-on experience with hospice patients. The emphasis on the curative aspects of medicine is coupled more with knowledge and skills for treating patients who are dying and beyond curing.

In addition to the development of hospice medical skills, training for medical personnel includes more in-depth exposure to multicultural values and traditions related to death and communication skills with diverse socioeconomic, multicultural, and other populations. The demographics of America are changing every day. Cultural diversity is not only here to stay, it is increasing faster than many perceive. This phenomenon must be dealt with appropriately if healthcare professionals are serious about success.

As I became more concerned about hospice patients and the elderly, I repeatedly came across data revealing major disparities in America's healthcare system. Overwhelming evidence indicates that these disparities negatively affect certain racial and ethnic groups. Health indicators for these affected groups impact the healthcare system and must be acknowledged and eliminated. America's long history of overt and covert racism, with all its stereotypes and discrimination, continues to pervade its institutions in ways underestimated by many people, including those who are victimized by it.

The Centers for Disease Control and Prevention confirms that wide racial and ethnic disparities persist in healthcare. Even when factors such as gender, condition, age, and socio-economic status are controlled, the inferior care is consistent across a range of illnesses and services.

The American Medical Association (AMA) also substantiates that racial and ethnic minorities still receive a lower quality of healthcare, resulting in higher death rates. The association's Program on Health Disparities and its Health Disparities Internal Working Group have developed the Recognition of Excellence in Eliminating Health Disparities program to educate and raise awareness on this issue.

If hospice care is to be embraced by racial and ethnic minorities, all barriers, particularly issues of culture and discrimination in healthcare, must be recognized and corrected. Many people of color have wounded hearts and valid reasons for harboring distrust for the healthcare system. One horrible reminder is the Tuskegee Institute Syphilis Experiment conducted with 399 African American men between 1932 and 1972 by the U.S. Public Health Service. Living in one of Alabama's poorest counties, these men, all in the late stages of syphilis, were mostly illiterate sharecroppers who trusted government doctors' offer of free treatment. Patients were never told they had syphilis. The men were allowed to degenerate with tumors, paralysis, heart disease, blindness, insanity, and death. Data for the experiment were collected from the men's autopsies, another fact that was concealed from them. The disease also infected many of their wives and children. In *Bad Blood: The Tuskegee Syphilis Experiment,* author James Jones refers to this experiment as "the longest non-therapeutic experiment on human beings in medical history."

Published in 2007, *Medical Apartheid: The Dark History of Medical Experimentation on Black Americans from Colonial Times to the Present* by Harriet A. Washington presents numerous documented examples of involuntary experimentation targeting African Americans, including those in military and prison environments. Some incidents occurred as late as the 1990s such as the injection of Fenfluramine into African American children in New York. Researchers investigating the genetic origins of violence used this drug. Further emphasizing racial and ethnic disparities, the author mentions abusive experimental research in Africa, Asia, and Latin America. Dying, particularly for people of color, has held hands with injustice too many times. It is little wonder that many regard the healthcare system with deep distrust.

The responsibility for changing attitudes that cause disparities within the healthcare system rests with that system. This is not only a healthcare issue, but also a moral one. This system cannot continue to sit down in the middle of an unjust road, cause harm to others, and not be held accountable. Healthcare providers must own the fact that a large amount of research on disparities in racial and ethnic minority healthcare is true and make every effort to demonstrate equitable practices.

Better education in racial and ethnic cultural sensitivity, however, is not enough. Negative stereotypes are activated with and without intent, particularly in high-pressure work environments. Serious accountability from healthcare providers must include rewards and penalties. Incentives should be offered to encourage healthcare institutions to work diligently at lowering their incidents of disparities against racial and ethnic minorities, as well as women and low economic groups. Solutions must be implemented with ongoing monitoring. Disparities of the magnitude that exists now will not be willed away.

The U.S. Department of Health and Human Services Council on Health Disparities was created to coordinate and unify Health and Human Services actions on issues related to health disparities among African Americans, Hispanics, Native Americans, Alaskan Natives, Asians, and Pacific Islanders. These groups are victimized by more death and diseases than the general population. Success of the council should improve the reduction in racial and ethnic health disparities.

The future of hospice must involve the participation of more racial and ethnic minorities at every level, particularly as patients. People view the world through their cultures and values. To ignore this fact and impose one's own culture and values on others caters to miscommunication and alienation. With respect and sensitivity, bridges can be built that help people connect at human levels, regardless of their differences. The availability of more language interpreters at healthcare institutions can facilitate this communication and bonding. Ongoing education on the culture and traditions of various populations, along with the understanding that varying beliefs exist within each group, must be increased throughout the healthcare system to improve service to diverse groups.

For example, many Latin Americans have a high regard for family responsibility in caregiving during the last stages of life. This may create reluctance on their part to seek help outside the family from a healthcare institution, even though this help could be beneficial, particularly as responsibilities increase. Because Hispanics are the largest ethnic minority in America, they need more hospice and palliative care outreach to assist them with providing loved ones with the extensive care they need. Effective strategies, which are sensitive to their culture, can be used to educate them on the availability and benefits of hospice support. Outreach should include dissemination of information, oral and written, via Spanish-language media used by the elderly, English-language media, churches, work sites, senior centers, schools, community centers, and other organizations. Community events can serve as outlets for outreach. Input from Latin Americans themselves is the best way to assess their needs and ways to address them.

Many Asian Americans also prefer family caregiving of their aging, dying relatives. In addition to being reluctant to place their elders in nursing homes for hospice care, they may also be reluctant to discuss specifics about illnesses with those in their care to keep them hopeful and without worry. Again, more knowledge of Asian American culture, including input from Asian Americans, should be gathered by healthcare providers in order to discover effective outreach procedures that expose Asian Americans to the beneficial possibilities of hospice support that are available to them.

Respect for racial, ethnic, and cultural diversity should be displayed in the aesthetics of healthcare institutions. That's another way to build trust, make the climate inviting for everyone, and send a message to the public about where the institutions stand in terms of diversity. What might seem like a small omission to others really isn't small at all. That's why input from diverse groups is so important when decisions that impact various populations are made. People tend to look for the familiar, for signs of themselves, their culture, when they find themselves in unfamiliar institutional settings. Pictures and other aesthetic touches that reflect diversity send powerful messages to the public. The message sent as a result of their absence is just as important as the message sent through their presence. Every person in the healthcare system must commit to real acceptance and respect, not just tolerance, of all people in the human family.

Another way to make this a reality is by adding more cultural diversity to the workforce of healthcare professions. While the demand for nurses and other medical personnel increases with the aging of the general population, the U.S. Department of Health and Human Services predicts the continuation of a major shortage of registered nurses in future years. The role of hospice volunteers will become even more important in delivering patient care. But hospice volunteers will not solve the shortage or diversity problems. Ongoing procedures must be implemented to retain current workers and recruit new ones. More bilingual recruits should be encouraged to enter healthcare professions.

Outreach in the business community, educational institutions, churches, and community organizations can play a significant role in educating the public and in recruiting diverse volunteers and potential employees. Older workers and displaced or retired workers from other industries should be considered. Many people would be willing to get involved if they were presented with an explanation of the crisis and the important role they can play in providing help.

Concerns related to improvements in the future of nursing homes and hospice care are numerous. Some problems involve uncontrollable variables, but those that can be controlled must be confronted. Fortunately, concerned advocates have already accepted the challenge to make improvements and are actively involved in implementing them. These people started wherever they happened to be. Many more advocates are needed to support efforts toward progress. Dr. Martin Luther King, Jr. said, "Take the first step in faith. You don't have to see the whole staircase, just take the first step."

Choosing Yes

Inside our minds,
possibilities pull us
like mighty waves
to explore new waters.
Mired in familiar floods,
we wade in the mundane,
soak in the safe,
distance ourselves from
life's problems lapping
at personal realities.
When we reach currents
between yes and no,
sound solutions surface.
Let's dare to dive in,
ride rivers of risks, swim
in the deepness of yes.

—Frances Shani Parker

15 School–Nursing Home Partnership

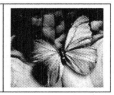

As an educator, I have observed that schools and nursing homes share many similarities. Both have climates or cultures that impact people in institutions. A paradigm shift in how these institutions are perceived, not only by the public, but also by those who work in the institutions, is long overdue. Roles of employees must be redefined. Teachers and administrators who work directly with students in schools should have more input in decision-making and receive more appreciation for what they do. Along those same lines, nursing home employees who give direct care to patients and know them best should have more input in patient care. They should feel more respected than many currently do.

People who enter schools and healthcare institutions like nursing homes should connect with a positive energy that heightens satisfaction in being there. Climates improve as institutions become more sensitive to employees' and constituents' needs. Ultimately, institutions are created by people, not by buildings or cosmetic changes.

On several occasions, I have been asked what my greatest achievement as an educator is, and I have always had a ready response. My greatest achievement as an educator is the composite of all the times I positively impacted lives. Everybody can positively impact lives on some level. The composite of all the improvements in quality of life for patients is the greatest achievement of employees in nursing homes.

In order for nursing homes and hospice care to fully enhance quality of life, patients must have experiences similar to what students need in schools. Patients must know that their progress as individuals with specialized needs is the primary motivation for everything that goes on in nursing homes. They must feel that their environments are safe, that trustworthy employees care about them and listen to them with their hearts.

Patients must know that the personal histories they bring to nursing homes are honored and that they will be encouraged to use their strengths in productive ways to improve their self-esteem and enhance the lives of others. They come to nursing homes with life stories that matter. Patients with dementia should be challenged to learn new skills in non-threatening ways. All patients' talents and accomplishments should be communicated to others.

Nursing home residents should be treated like the adults they are. They need to have more input regarding scheduling and other decisions about their lives. Patients who are terminally ill may not want to wake up at the same time every day with three sick roommates snoring, screaming, or talking to themselves. Finally, patients must be confident that caregivers and medical personnel support their efforts to leave with dignity. Dying is a form of "graduation." It is the culmination of a life and should be treated with great respect.

Like a school faculty, nursing home employees must be trained well and held to high standards of accountability in performing their assigned duties. Consistent monitoring by supervisors who are also monitored should be the norm. Monitoring should be documented and used to evaluate performance. Systems of rewards and penalties should be implemented and enforced consistently. Expressions of staff appreciation should be ongoing, immediate if time permits, or in writing whenever possible. Input from all levels of workers and constituents should be encouraged. There should be a team atmosphere in which everyone's contributions count.

In a school environment, knowledge of best practices gives everyone an achievable vision that has been proven successful. Best practices of nursing homes around the country and abroad should be systematically disseminated to all nursing homes. There is a great need for information about nursing homes that use hospice and palliative care effectively and those that emphasize patient-centered care. Nursing homes that have integrated hospice care well into their programs should serve as models for others that need assistance. Opportunities to network at local levels, nationwide, and globally should be promoted on a larger scale.

Schools and nursing homes have a natural bond among their constituents. As a child, I had the good fortune of having regular contact with both my grandmother and great grandmother. No doubt, they are partially responsible for my concern with the elderly. I especially remember my great grandmother really listening to what I had to say, and I had plenty to say. Elderly people often have a patient wisdom that only comes with living a long life. Relationships between children and the elderly should be encouraged more. The unique exchanges that take place in this context are lacking too often in today's society.

The most effective learning usually does not come from classroom lectures or always translate on standardized tests. I witnessed academic and affective growth by students as a direct result of their interactions with the elderly when the two groups became involved in meaningful projects such as letter writing, storytelling, biography writing, arts and crafts, and performing arts. This excellent educational approach to teaching and learning that connects classroom learning with meeting community needs is called service-learning. A growing body of research shows that students derive many benefits in areas of academic achievement, enthusiasm for learning, caring for others, and greater civic and political engagement through involvement in service-learning.

When I was a teacher, I took children on service-learning field trips to nursing homes. Students practiced educational skills, showcased their talents, and provided entertainment and companionship to residents. These trips came about after extensive student preparation and included ongoing reflection and evaluation of growth. Some children feared the elderly, particularly those in nursing home settings. They also believed several negative stereotypes about the elderly such as their being grouchy and sad. Many people do not embrace the elderly as positive contributors to society or as engaging social beings. Children learn this early in life. Then adults complain when children don't respect their elders.

During one of my first nursing home visits with fifth graders, we experienced an incident that made me grateful I had prepared students well before the visit. As we walked down the hall to leave the nursing home, a woman in a wheelchair reached out for my hand. I thought she wanted to shake it, so I let her hold it. With a firm grip on my hand, she proceeded to lick it. When she finished, she graciously let go and grinned widely, meaning no harm. During this teachable moment, my students watched my reaction. Children study and learn from behaviors of all adults with whom they have contact. I responded normally. We had already discussed beforehand that some residents might act in an unusual manner because they were ill. We told the woman goodbye with calmness and respect. I headed for a bathroom to vigorously wash my hand.

After our return to school, my students reflected on this incident in a detailed discussion about what occurred. "Dementia" was included as one of their vocabulary words. It wasn't a word in their textbooks or on their standardized tests, but they had experienced its meaning firsthand and expanded their information about the complex human mind. Service-learning projects benefited seniors and increased students' knowledge about nursing homes, aging, illness, and dying.

"Hello, Ms. Wokie. My name is Xavier. My class came today to visit you and other people at this nursing home. We've been looking forward to coming back here. Today, we're going to sing some new songs we learned and read a few poems we wrote. We've been working on writing poetry at school."

"Xavier, singing songs and writing poems sound great. I used to write poems when I was growing up. I even recited one at my church in front of the whole congregation. Everybody clapped and made me feel special. This should be a really nice program."

"I sure hope it is. I don't know if you remember me from my last visit here. This time, I have on a red shirt, instead of a brown one like the last time. My teacher said I'm your partner today."

"You know, I think I do remember you. What I really remember is that you had on those eyeglasses. I wear eyeglasses, too."

"Oh, you do wear glasses, just like me! Did people ever tease you about wearing glasses? Sometimes I get called "four-eyed.""

"Isn't that something? I used to get called "four-eyed" when I was a girl. But I didn't let those kids get to me. I knew I needed my glasses, so I could see what the teacher wrote on the blackboard and read my books. I wasn't going to let some kids teasing me keep me from doing my best. Don't pay them any mind. I bet you'll do better than a lot of those kids who tease you. Besides, what's wrong with having two extra eyes?"

"You're funny, Ms. Wokie! I'll remember that when they tease me again. My glasses do make my reading better. I love to read."

"That's good. I do, too. I started that habit when I was young, just like you. It's one of the best things I ever did. We didn't have a lot of books, but that didn't stop me from reading everything I could get my hands on, especially comic books and newspapers. Reading is what made me decide to become a secretary. I had to read and type a lot. Have you been thinking much about what you want to be when you grow up? Time is slow when you're young, but one day you'll be all grown up and taking care of yourself."

"I think about being a bunch of things. Right now, I want to be an actor, a doctor, and a basketball player.

Some people say that's silly to want to be all those things. But I like them all and can't make up my mind on one."

"I don't think that's silly at all. Those jobs are good honest ways to make a living. Son, you just keep on getting your education and thinking about living your dreams. The main thing is to have dreams. Whatever you decide to be, pick a job you really like that makes you happy. Do your best. If you're happy doing your job, you'll feel like you're getting paid to have fun most of the time."

"Then I won't mind getting up every day to go to work. Oh-oh, looks like it's almost time for our show to start. I have to go up to the stage with my class. I'm going to come on third. I'm not as nervous as I was the last time I came here. But I still hope I don't mess up."

"Baby, you're going to do just fine. You already did something nice just by coming here to spend time with us. Time is one of the greatest gifts you can give somebody."

"After the show, Ms. Wokie, I'll push your wheelchair over to the refreshments table. We can eat together and talk some more. I have a list of questions to ask you about your life. I'm going to write a story about you when I go back to school. My class is making a big book with stories about all our nursing home partners. Everybody here will get a copy when it's finished. That way you can find out more about other people here, and they can learn more about you."

"A story about my life, imagine that! That's wonderful! I'd love to have refreshments with you, Xavier. I want to hear more about your life, too. You know, I liked you the minute I laid my four eyes on you."

Laughing while skipping away, Xavier responds, "Got to go now! See you in a little while!"

When students returned to school, there was always plenty to discuss during our reflection time. Everybody had something special to share about impressions of the elderly. Students mentioned how residents seemed to enjoy being around them, how those with dementia responded enthusiastically to their singing, even though they fell asleep sometimes. Students were reminded again that people with strange behaviors are still worthy of kindness and respect because they are part of that huge flower garden called the human family. "Diversity" joined other cool words on their growing vocabulary list. They wrote about their experiences in their journals, drew pictures, and created skits about what they had seen. They even made up a few rap songs that they performed to the delight of their nursing home friends on a return visit.

Because they had completed a survey they created before the trip, the students were amazed to see how wrong some of their assumptions were when they took the same survey after we returned. They seemed surprised that elderly people had lead vibrant lives and were still interesting people. They were fascinated by similarities they shared when the elderly talked about their childhood adventures. It never occurred to students that people who were so much older than they were could understand their feelings and opinions or care so much about them. They displayed their survey results on graphs with trip pictures, so others could see the exciting conclusions of their research. And they improved their academic skills throughout the entire project.

The beauty of service-learning is that it can be integrated into any school curriculum in all subject areas and grade levels, including special education classes. All it takes is willing teachers finding interesting ways to match learning requirements with meeting community needs. Plants studied in a science class can easily be grown and donated to recipients who can benefit from them nutritionally. Practicing their required sorting skills while using different toiletries such as toothbrushes and soap, preschool, learning-disabled students can create gift baskets for homeless people. Appropriate matches are endless. Supportive administrators, parents, community, and business people enhance the affective and academic impact of this teaching-learning approach.

Many high schools and colleges seek potential service recipients such as nursing home residents, so students can interact positively with the elderly, complete school service requirements, develop leadership skills, and learn about possible careers. My first volunteer experience in a nursing home was as a high school student involved in a service organization. To this day, applesauce reminds me of a woman I used to feed then. No doubt, other insights remain with me regarding that experience. I had no idea then that I would still be volunteering at nursing homes many years later. This kind of exposure builds character and reinforces values promoting good citizenship. Students don't always receive these motivations at home. Service to others reflects well on both high school and college transcripts. Schools and nursing homes should implement more partnerships through service-learning.

Major institutionalized changes often meet with resistance, but change can come after persistent efforts. Years ago, keeping nursing home residents restrained, even when they were immobile, was considered nurturing and protective. Just as widespread corporal punishment in schools was viewed as necessary to discipline students, keeping patients restrained in wheelchairs was deemed acceptable behavior for nursing homes. Unfortunately, restrained patients became weak and developed sores.

Nurses led the movement for replacing practices of restraint by suggesting alternative methods that gave patients more freedom. Growing bodies of research supported their cause, and the negative practices declined. Many people were resistant to those changes, and some still are. But those practices of the past violate laws and are not condoned by most institutions. According to federal law, patient restraints can only be used now when ordered by a doctor as part of a patient's medical treatment.

Common bonds between schools and nursing homes can be used creatively to enhance the lives of students and nursing home residents. Many people say, "It takes a whole village to raise a child." With the implementation of service-learning partnerships between schools and nursing homes, everyone involved in service learning wins. It takes a whole village to make a village whole.

Student Reflections

I know you forget
you have a roommate,
imagine you take distant trips,
see me as a short brown blur
when I visit your nursing home.

I know your childhood
friends whisper secrets,
your favorite dress has ruffles,
my cards touch you with sunshine,
you love the stories I tell.

I know that carrots
make you frown,
my visits swing you higher,
loneliness glues you down,
you miss your friends who died.

I know you teach me
about new things,
praise me when I'm good,
help me care about others
the way you care about me.

—Frances Shani Parker

16 Baby Boomer Haven

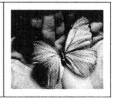

Welcome to Baby Boomer Haven! It's a treasure to have you. My name is Ruth, and I'll be your tour guide today. The first thing you need to know about our nursing home is that it's real for some, but imaginary for too many others. Everything we enjoy here already exists in nursing homes scattered throughout America, but not in nearly enough. We're having this tour today, so you can become familiar with possibilities that all nursing home residents should be experiencing in culture change, no matter where they are located. When baby boomers seeking institutional healthcare show up in the millions, nursing homes like ours should be ready to receive them with welcoming lights shining in every window. Now, more than ever, nursing homes should be focused on ongoing state-of-the-art improvements. The comfortable life we live is as close as society's handshake with commitment to quality healthcare, particularly for the ill and elderly.

We love many things about living here, but what we enjoy most is that we're treated with dignity as adults. Our feelings and opinions matter. You'll understand this better during the tour when you see our physical environment, the freedom we have in deciding how we live within our limitations, and the nurturing manner in which all employees interact with us.

Before we start, let me give you a little background about our home. Our energy-efficient building is designed with divisions called houses with "families" consisting of smaller units of residents and permanent staff. Houses provide specialized patient care from certified employees. We have one hundred medically assessed residents here in long-term care, short-term rehabilitation, and short-term terminal care known as hospice care. Staff and residents had input in the design of our home.

We receive a full range of medical services, including palliative care for patients who are chronically ill. In addition, we have dental, psychiatric, speech, and hearing services. Most rooms are single, but double rooms with privacy areas for meeting with visitors and being alone are available for those who prefer them. All rooms have bathrooms. We have a childcare center, too. Residents, employees, and children benefit greatly from this component. Diversity is celebrated here, and we are always encouraged to come together and share as a community. This is our home. It belongs to us.

But I've talked enough. Let's get this party started. If you follow my wheelchair balloon, you won't get lost. We'll stay together during the tour. There'll be plenty of time later for you to explore the many sights and activities that interest you, including one of our first-class dining rooms where buffet dinners are served daily. We'll start outside with the friendly face of where we live.

Although we are located in the heart of a big city, we still love to see nature dressed up in all her glory. Did you know research studies show that contact with nature can improve a person's mental health and even lower blood pressure? I love sitting in my rocking chair out here on the front porch surrounded by nature. It reminds me of when I used to sit on the porch getting my hair combed down South when I was a girl. That's where I heard grownups tell stories about my family and African American history. The front porch is where I first grabbed a handle on life. In later years, that was where my own children learned life lessons and heard stories that were passed down through generations. Nowadays, other residents and I rock our chairs to discussions about everything imaginable. Don't get me started on some of the far-out things we talk about, and age doesn't have a thing to do with it.

Our outdoor landscape, which includes walking paths, stays well maintained. The park area with the playground equipment and picnic benches is where the children play. Sometimes we eat outside at the tables when we have barbecues. Our "families" also have courtyard areas where we can socialize outdoors. Those of us who enjoy gardening like to participate in the upkeep of the grounds. Some of us had to leave gardens when we moved here, so it's good to continue our hobby. We have a communal garden in the back where we grow vegetables, and a lovely greenhouse on the roof. Our green thumbers are kept busy. If you think outside looks pretty, wait until you see how Mother Nature has taken up residence inside.

We have parking available both underground and above ground. All visitors who enter our premises are screened and monitored. Some guests say they come by to visit residents more often, especially at night, because they feel more secure. Monitored video cameras are strategically stationed outdoors and throughout the building to help everybody feel safe.

Transportation is another area in which we try to be sensitive to needs of residents and family members. Some families are not able to use public transportation to visit loved ones on a regular basis. Outpatient care is also difficult for some to receive when reliable transportation is not available. We provide vans to transport residents and family members whenever they need this assistance. We also use this service to allow eligible residents to take short personal trips.

We have a cyberspace home at our website. Family members can view their loved ones over the Internet in certain areas of the nursing home and see what they're doing. These innovations resulted from decisions made by our Baby Boomer Council, which consists of resident, employee, family, and community representatives. We also have house councils and "family" meetings where we do what I call "praising and preaching" when we celebrate one another and address any concerns we have. We invite everybody's input in decision-making and post signs inside that say, "Help us help you." Speaking of inside, let's go there now and see what's happening.

Watch out for Diva Dog over there, one of several resident pets. She's just looking you over to make sure you look her over. In her spare time, she's a certified psychologist. For patients who prefer the convenience of a responsive robotic pet, we have two mechanical dogs that operate with artificial intelligence. They provide playful companionship without the need for feeding, walking, and cleaning up after them. The best part about the mechanical dogs is that the more patients interact with them, the more responsive the dogs become to the patients. All the animals here are like our extended family, and for some of us, they are family. Other indoor animals on the site are located in our aviaries of brightly colored birds and in our aquariums with fish that mesmerize us with their antics. We have more animals outdoors such as horses and rabbits. It's fascinating watching how all of our animals relate. They're a lot like people, you know, and have much more sense than we think they do.

You could call this first room our communal living room, instead of a lobby, because the fireplace, comfortable furniture, plants, and homelike atmosphere are so inviting. Our smaller houses have living rooms, too. Notice the murals of street scenes that make us feel like we're strolling in a real neighborhood. We even have an espresso bar where we can sit on a park bench and have something to drink. As we continue walking, we pass our beauty shop, game room, chapel, and library. Carpeted floors make falling down a lot less painful, and the wall railings give us something to grip when we want to take walks. Exercise is so important. Rest areas along the route give those who need a break a place to talk, read, or just refuel.

We're encouraged to personalize our rooms as much as possible. That's why our rooms and doors are decorated to reflect our taste. This is my room, I have blue flowered curtains that my daughter made especially for me. Every day, I awaken to an expression of her love. I enjoy sewing for her, too. We know each other by heart. Residents can use certain furniture we brought from our homes. That chair has been in my family for many years.

That's Erika's room with the Jewish symbols on the door. She's a Holocaust survivor who has many historically rich stories to tell. Erika survived childhood because a family sympathetic to the plight of Jews hid her for years. She still recalls the choking fear that gripped her during the times she heard soldiers' voices outside. Some people in the world still want to believe that the Holocaust never happened. If you know people like that, tell them to come talk to Erika. Her first-hand testimony and pictures give history a name with a living person. She reminds us about creating a better future.

This is Stone Sequoyah's room. On his door, he likes to use Native American symbols and stories to celebrate his culture. Because of him, I know about the Trail of Tears, the white buffalo story, and fascinating Native American customs. Did you know that many African Americans developed positive bonds with Native Americans who helped them when they escaped during U.S. slavery? I learn and appreciate a lot about people just by walking through the halls and checking out their doors. It certainly keeps me busy on my walks.

This might be a little unusual, but I just have to show you one of our bathing rooms. We have choices about whether we want a shower, a bath, or a sponge bath and when we choose to take them. The Jacuzzi tubs and music are great motivators to come here. Deodorizers keep our bathrooms smelling fresh at all times. Notice the bright artwork that colors the walls and even the ceilings, so we can admire beauty when we are in reclining positions. We can soak in beauty everywhere we look. These simple touches tell us that somebody thought we were worth the effort.

Speaking of pictures on the walls, I know you've noticed action pictures of residents, employees, and visitors on the walls. We enjoy displaying memories of our good times together as a community. If you look over to your right, you'll see one of several "We Did It!" boards highlighting accomplishments of residents and employees. For staff and patients who are able to leave our home, we include information and pictures about their lives away from home. We know who sings in the choir, what their hobbies are, about their trips, and general news about their families. We're always looking for opportunities to be standing ovations for one another. Every other month we have a talent show with employees and residents performing. We look forward to learning more about our caregivers and resident neighbors.

The other great pictures you see on display are artwork created by local school children. Every month, a school sends a group to decorate an area with items students made. Sometimes the decorations are seasonal, but many times they reflect the students' creativity relating to subjects they are learning in school. Occasionally, they display information and pictures about field trips they have taken. During the fall season, many students visit apple orchards and farms. We love to see their pictures capturing rural scenes that are so rare in the city. Viewing their projects on different countries, where some of us have traveled or even lived, provides many hours of interesting information and conversation.

Our weekly "Baby Boomer Business" newsletter is another vehicle we use for spreading good news about everyone here, including our animals. Some residents have their articles, stories, and poems published in the newsletter. We learn facts from the past that help us understand one another better. For example, Edna knows all about foreign countries because she used to be a worldwide travel agent. Reports from various committees keep us aware of what's going on now and in the future here. We make sure residents' families get copies of our newsletter, so they can keep track of all the activities to which they are invited to join us. I guess I should warn you that Nosy, our calico cat over there, has his own gossip column. Be careful what you say around him. You never know when he's eavesdropping. Bless his heart.

Employees seem to love working here as much as we love living here. Most have years of seniority, and hardly anybody is ever absent. Low staff turnover saves considerable money in overtime and in hiring temporary help. Two things all employees like are our flexible scheduling and community childcare on the premises. This allows them to personalize their time and accomplish more at home and at work with fewer worries. If you look to your left through the window of the childcare center, you can see two employees having lunch with their children. The older gentleman is a resident reading to a small group. I love spending time with the little ones. I jokingly call them my little "ankle biters" when they aren't around. Some of them call me, "Grandma," and a few like to say "Big Mama," which really tickles me because that's what I called my grandmother.

Management and staff have a great working relationship. Together they wrap us in a warm family quilt woven with reassurance. Everybody participates in decision-making and attends workshops, classes, and conferences to keep abreast of best practices in their fields. Various staff members and residents are included in the hiring of new employees and, when appropriate, involved in their training. Periodic meetings are held with all shifts represented, so more in-depth information can be provided concerning patients. Employees take pride in their work and strive to continue our tradition of excellence. We're all part of the same team, and we're all cheerleaders.

It's wonderful having nurse aides we like on a regular basis. Nurse aides or CNAs are the people who give us daily hands-on care, the people with whom we communicate and spend time with most. Their workloads and pay are reasonable, and they feel confident that they will succeed. Like other employees, their input is welcome. All of our new nurse aides are mentored and evaluated by experienced nurses before they are allowed to work independently. This helps the new nurse aides learn how to respond to our needs and practice correct skills from the very beginning. Morale stays high because they feel empowered. They know their contributions are important and appreciated.

Residents enjoy plenty of flexibility, too. As we approach this dining area, keep in mind that we have several small homelike dining rooms to encourage socialization among residents. Also, each house has its own kitchen where small dishes can be prepared and made available at all times. We wake up and eat on our own schedules. I don't know how some people can part their eyelids at 5:30 AM when breakfast starts. I like my breakfast around 9:30 AM when my engine begins to purr.

We choose from two or three entrees and desserts, when available, for each meal. Our menus are creative, varied, and enjoyable. Occasionally, we even sample dishes using a favorite recipe of a resident. That's always a tasty surprise. Residents participate on the food committee and give suggestions. We sample new foods before they are included on the regular menus. Most of us just want simple meals and a little background music.

Those residents who are able can select food from a buffet in this dining room. Believe me, when we make our own salads and pour gravy on our own mashed potatoes like Valerie is doing over there, we know we're in charge. It's amazing how so few residents here have weight-loss problems.

Sometimes we have theme dinners that celebrate hobbies, songs, and different countries. We always have healthy snacks available. Family members and friends are welcome to join us during meals and celebrations such as birthday parties, Mardi Gras balls, and even weddings. Yes, old folks fall in love and get married, too. Many of us love good dance music. Don't think for one minute that we can't still shake what our mamas gave us.

Do you feel how calm it is walking through our home? That's because you don't hear a PA system calling employees to do something every three minutes. Technology plays an important role here in patient care. All of our employees wear emergency electronic devices to maintain voice contact with other staff members. Patients' call bells are connected to employee personal digital assistants (PDAs) to provide immediate assistance.

All information about patients is computerized, secure, and easily available to medical personnel. This includes patients' advanced directives, which can always be updated at their request, and ongoing evaluations about pain that can be addressed quickly. A state-of-the-art wireless computer network keeps track of where patients are at all times.

Electronic devices worn by patients convey real-time vital signs to a computer and can be used to contact nurses. Wheelchairs brake automatically and include alarms for pads, seatbelt buckles, and cushions. Bathroom sensors alert nurses if patients fall. We have an electronic database on all falls that includes date, time, place, location, and any other pertinent information that can help us prevent falls in the future.

Touch-screen computers allow nurse aides to input assessment information about patients. Voice recognition is also available for inputting information. Bar-code medication administration increases patient safety. Wireless and mobile computer capabilities provide patient information that can be accessed by doctors from secure locations outside the nursing home such as a hospital. We like the use of technology because it gives employees more time for "nursing" us at home.

We're about to pass a few of our multipurpose activity and therapy rooms. Our fitness pool and whirlpools are also located in this area. Oh, look! Several of our ladies with "hatitude" are having their monthly Red Hat Hotties meeting. There's no telling what fun activity that feisty group might be planning. Because they're senior citizens, they say they've earned the right to do whatever they feel like doing. They presented a fantastic "Bewitching Beachwear" fashion show last summer. Involvement in various activities stimulates and challenges us mentally and physically. We keep busy with games, arts and crafts, woodworking, writing, acting, dancing, reading, storytelling, and singing. We take field trips to restaurants, malls, ball games, special events, and theaters. Everyone who is able to participate is welcome. Sometimes we go on outings with just the members of our houses or "families," so we can bond more as small communities.

Activities are available all day and during evenings on a daily basis. This practice is especially important for patients who experience what is called "sundowning," an energy burst that some patients get around sundown between 6:00 and 8:00 in the evening. Without monitored outlets for these energy outbursts, some patients could be injured through falls. Patients can become more confused and combative during these periods. Appropriate therapeutic activities such as games, singing, and reading, protect residents while keeping them entertained.

Many residents are involved in recreational therapy, occupational therapy, physical therapy, and relearning life skills. We even have therapy sessions to improve muscle tone with horseback riding in our equestrian program. The first time I ever rode a horse was right here on the grounds of this nursing home. I was seventy-five years young. What a thrill that was sitting high on my horse for real!

Each floor has a lounge area where we can get together with our friends and have a good time doing what we call our "gossiping and playing-games therapy." Our days are definitely exciting and full. But just to make sure that we're all mellow, residents are screened regularly for depression.

At Baby Boomer Heaven, I mean Haven, we emphasize win-win community service. When we join with the community and put all of our notes together, we create some fine songs. Of course, we appreciate service from others, but we want to serve people, too. We want to feel like we are doing our part to make the world a better place now and for future generations.

Our gift shop sells crafts we make to help fund service projects. Among several services we provide, residents help Fetching Feasts provide meals delivered to seniors at their homes. We perform tasks here that make the process easier for them. We also sew blankets for newborns and tutor and read to children at our childcare center. In addition to calling shut-ins who live alone, we also call to check on latchkey children of families who know us well and want their children to have that extra support when adults aren't home. Sometimes we help children with homework problems or advise them about typical social problems with friends. Letters and e-mails are exchanged regularly with our elementary school pen pals. Their teachers say the students seem more excited about writing when they know real people will respond to what they have to say. We also allow schools and other community groups to use our auditorium for meetings and special programs.

We especially enjoy serving our local community because they are our neighbors who have been very good to us. University faculty members and students partner with us for research projects that will ultimately help other senior citizens. They also lead interesting discussion classes about current events, government programs, and other topics that stimulate our minds and keep us informed. Several organizations, churches, and businesses have become official partners. They send volunteers here on a regular basis to assist in any way they can. We keep lists detailing our needs gathered through resident and employee surveys. We let volunteers select how they can help us. We have meetings with them to be sure we all understand and agree in writing about service projects. These steps are important because those who perform service should never assume they know other people's needs. Sometimes volunteers suggest a service that's not on our list, and the idea turns out to be a winner. But we still discuss and agree before implementing. That's what happened when manicures were donated by the beauty salon down the street. Check out the butterflies on my nails.

Our partners help us with fundraising by donating money, equipment, and expertise to support many of our activities and trips. One company copies all of our newsletters for us. We give them a free ad in the newsletter to thank them. Another company has assisted many of us in developing computer skills. Now, some of us make our own websites, email relatives and friends often, and teach what we've learned to other residents. A restaurant donates the refreshments for our annual intergenerational dance when the high school students come and twirl us on the dance floor. Students enjoy doing the twist as much as we did when we were young. We also dance in our wheelchair hustle line. We love to recognize and honor all of our volunteers at an annual luncheon. They truly do make a positive difference in our lives, and they say we make one in theirs.

If you think the floor plan in this house where we are currently walking is a little different from previous houses, you're right. This house belongs to patients with forms of dementia such as Alzheimer's disease. We try not to let this house get too noisy or confusing for them. The floor plan is designed to ease disorientation of these residents as they explore their surroundings. The path they follow is circular with no dead ends to frustrate them. This makes it easier for them to stay focused.

Along the route, are resting places with games, catalogs, magazines, and an aquarium. In case there is a need to refocus an aggressive patient's attention, there are wall distractions such as bells and lights that staff members can use. Landmarks and pictograms are used as reference points. Posted signs are easy to understand. Patients can readily see places or activities that might interest them like this lovely glass-enclosed patio where they can socialize with others, including patients from other houses, and observe birds in the aviary surrounded with flowers.

Our residents with dementia get expert medical care, along with touch and massage therapy with aromatherapy. Staff members give them special attention, using techniques that help them feel confident. Keeping them comfortable and safe are major priorities. Because dementia is progressive, predictions about how patients will behave each day, based on what they've done in the past, are not always accurate. While we have superior security throughout our facility, patients in this house are enrolled in the Safe-Return Protection Program sponsored by the Alzheimer's Association. They all wear identification bracelets and clothing labels that provide 24-hour assistance for them via a national phone number in case they ever wander or become lost outside this building. This is especially comforting on trips with us or family members. Even the most careful plans can go awry, but this program supports the behavior of persons with dementia.

Diversionary and calming activities such as using rocking chairs, carrying a doll or something else to hold, fold, or squeeze are helpful to them. Their names and pictures are on their room doors, which vary in color to help them distinguish their rooms from others. Their rooms often display familiar furniture, photographs, and other objects from the past. They also have recordings of their favorite songs and stories, along with DVDs of movies they like. Relatives and friends are encouraged to visit often to interact with them. Staff members suggest interactive activities when visitors need assistance.

Our last stop is the hospice house. Everyone has private rooms large enough to accommodate a daybed for caregivers who need to rest during the day or stay overnight. Dedicated volunteers, including a few employees, are assigned to be present with dying patients who have no one to stay with them during the final stage of their death journey. A few hospice patients who can still get around also volunteer to be with other hospice patients. Volunteers provide welcome respite for caregivers who need time away from their many responsibilities. We support our caregivers by giving them baskets with donated items such as toiletries, writing materials, snacks and drinks. We try to accommodate them with any available items or services that we can, including the use of computers and music players.

Medical personnel trained in hospice and palliative care, including pain management, are available at all times. A multi-disciplined pressure sore prevention program helps to maintain patients' comfort. Sensitivity to patients' values and cultures is the norm. Everyone who works here honors the death journey. This is not a rule. It's a philosophy that we live every day. An added benefit is that implementing the hospice philosophy in our nursing home has made an important contribution toward the positive atmosphere and patient care throughout the nursing home. Best practices in one area have a way of influencing other areas.

Serenity permeates everything that goes on here. Many of our hospice patients enjoy music therapy to help soothe them through various stages of their illnesses. Harp music can be especially comforting. One of our community partners finances a "Wishing Well" project for hospice patients by making a wish come true for them. Recently, a patient had a special visit from a close friend with whom he had lost track for many years. The friend's trip was financed through the "Wishing Well" project. Two days after the heartwarming reunion, the patient died. At the family's request, the hospice chaplain coordinated a memorial service held here in our chapel. I was one of many who paid my respects to that kind gentleman.

It's hard to believe we're at the end of our tour already. There are many more wonderful things to say about our home. We're always finding new ways to update what we do. We hope you had a good time and that you learned more about quality nursing home and hospice care. Our elderly and ill deserve to be treated admirably. While we may appear to be old and worn, our hearts are wrinkle-free. Hopefully, knowing that everything you witnessed here today is already a reality in some nursing homes will encourage more creative solutions for improving the state of nursing homes across America.

On a personal note, I want you to know that I have been diagnosed as terminally ill. The hospice house is where I live now. As you can see, my mind is still finely tuned, but physically I can't get around much without my wheelchair anymore. Each week, I feel a little weaker, but I'm determined to suck the marrow of life from each day. Like many people, I never thought I would spend my last days in a nursing home, but here I am. And you know what? I'm happy with that. We're all going to die one day, and I'm prepared to take my turn. I live in great surroundings where dedicated hospice workers have made it possible for me to breathe the fresh air of contentment.

I want you to have a beautiful death like the one I'm expecting, a death experienced as a perfect parade of pleasant moments. We all know death's time, place, and circumstances are unpredictable. One day, you will reach a clearing almost on the Other Side of Through. If you're receiving hospice care in a nursing home somewhere, I hope it will be like this one or better. Most of all, I hope you will be at peace, maybe like a cocooned caterpillar anticipating butterflying good times later.

Reflections of a Hospice Volunteer

I leave my car and walk into a world with many fates.
The people live reality where three words dominate:
"Nostalgia" brings memories that make them question why.
"Delusions" create fantasies that often come alive.
"Anticipation" beckons the beginning of each day.
A visit, party, special news—what is on the way?

Sedonia tells me stories of how life used to be.
Many things seem different now. She's almost ninety-three.
Moochie shields unseen friends he pledges to protect.
I wonder if he sees and hears the friends he manifests.

Dexter smiles and says with pride while waiting for his son,
"All my children visit me, and each is Number One."
Pearl yells, "I want some cake, and bring it just for me!"
She thinks that I'm employed here. She sees me every week.

An empty bed reminds me that someone else has gone.
Next week, I'll see someone new. Life's cycle will go on.
Juan trails me through each room while planning his escape.
"I have somewhere to go," he pleads. I stop him at the gate.

I leave this special world today with wisdom strong and rare,
Respecting every circumstance that brought each person there.
Our futures are unknown to us like roads with endless curves.
I drive away feeling good, happy that I served.

                                              Frances Shani Parker

Ten Tips for
Becoming Dead Right

1. Accept death as part of life.

2. Listen to the universe.

3. Expect rainbow smiles.

4. Live a healthy lifestyle.

5. Be informed and proactive.

6. Do your best.

7. Give service to others.

8. Be grateful for blessings.

9. Put death wishes in writing.

10. Have a dignified death journey.

About the Author

Frances Shani Parker is a writer, consultant, and hospice volunteer. Her writing has won awards from *Writer's Digest*, the Poetry Society of Michigan, the Detroit Writer's Guild, Broadside Press, and the New Orleans Public Library. Among publications including her work are *Black Arts Quarterly* (Stanford University), *Warpland: A Journal of Black Literature and Ideas* (Chicago State University), *Voices of the Civil Rights Movement* (AARP), and two United Nations *Dialogue Through Poetry Anthology* e-books. Among venues at which her poems have been read are the International AIDS Conference in South Africa and "Artists Among Us," sponsored by the Michigan Wayne County Council for Arts, History, and Humanities.

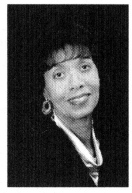

A former school principal, Parker has had essays and poems published in the educational arena, particularly on service learning, which is a teaching and learning method that connects classroom learning with meeting community needs. She has been honored with the Service-Learning Trailblazer Award presented by the National Service-Learning Partnership. Other honors include the Outstanding Educational Administrator Award presented by the Metropolitan Detroit Alliance of Black School Educators, and the Educator of the Year Award presented by the Wayne State University Chapter of Phi Delta Kappa, an international, professional fraternity for educators.

Parker's website is www.FrancesShaniParker.com.

Bibliography

Baker, B. (2007). *Old age in a new age: The promise of transformative nursing homes.* Nashville, TN: Vanderbilt University Press.

Berman, C. (2005). *Caring for yourself while caring for your aging parents: How to help, how to survive.* 3rd Edition. New York, NY: Owl Books

Carlson, E. & Hsiao, K. (2006). *The baby boomer's guide to nursing home care.* Lanham, MD: Taylor Trade Publishing.

Delehanty, H. & Ginzler, E., (2006). *Caring for your parents: The complete AARP guide.* New York, NY: Sterling Publishing Company, Inc.

Fairview Health Services, (1999). *The family handbook of hospice.* Minneappolis, MN: Fairview Press.

Green, C. R., Tait, R.C., & Gallagher, R.M. (Jan./Feb. 2005). The unequal burden of pain: disparities and differences. *Pain Medicine.* 6, 1-2.

Glenner, J. A., Stehman, J. M., Davagnino, J., Galante, M. J. & Green, M. L. (2005). *When your loved one has dementia.* Baltimore, MD: The John Hopkins University Press.

Jennings, B., True, R., D'Onofrio, C., & Baily. M. A. (Mar./Apr. 2003). Access to hospice care: expanding boundaries, overcoming barriers. *Hastings Center Report Special Supplement* 33. S53-S56.

Jones, J. H. (1991). Bad blood: *The tuskegee syphillis experiment.* Chicago, IL: African American Images.

Kay, C. B. (2003). *The complete guide to service learning: Proven, practical ways to engage students in civic responsibility, academic curriculum, & social action.* Minneapolis, MN: Free Spirit Publishing.

Kielsmeier, J., Neal, M. & Crossley, A. (2006). *Growing to greatness: The state of service-learning project.* Saint Paul, MN: State Farm Companies Foundation.

Kubler-Ross, E. (1997). *Questions and answers on death and dying.* New York, NY: First Touchstone Edition.

Lieberman, T. (2000). *Consumer reports complete guide to health services for seniors:* New York, NY: Three Rivers Press.

Noel, B. & Blair, P. D., (2003). *Living with grief: A guide for your first year of grieving.* Fredonia, WI: Champion Press, Ltd.

Palermo, M.T. & Edelman, R., (2004). *AARP crash course in estate planning: The essential guide to wills, trusts and your personal legacy* (AARP). New York, NY: Sterling Publishing Company, Inc.

Smedley, B.D, Stith, A.Y. & Nelson, A.R, (2003). *Unequal treatment: Confronting racial and ethnic disparities in health care.* Washington, DC: National Academies Press.

U.S. Department of Veterans Affairs, (2003). *Federal benefits for veterans and dependents.* Washington, DC: U.S. Department of Veteran Affairs.

U.S. General Accounting Office, (2003). GAO-03-561 *Nursing home quality: Prevalence of serious problems, while declining, reinforces importance of enhanced oversight.* Washington, D C: U. S. General Accounting Office.

Washington, H.A, (2007) *Medical apartheid: The dark history of medical experimentation on black americans from colonial times to the present.* New York, NY: Doubleday.

Worden, J.W. (2001) *Children and grief: When a parent dies.* New York, NY: The Guilford Press.

York, S. (2000). *Remembering well: rituals for celebrating life and mourning death.* San Francisco, CA: Jossey-Bass, Inc.

Resources

AARP, 601 E Street NW, Washington, DC 20049; Tel. (888)-OUR-AARP (888)-687-2277); www.aarp.org

Alzheimer's Association National Office, 225 N. Michigan Avenue, 17th Floor, Chicago, IL 60601; Tel. (800) 272-3900; www.alz.org

American Academy of Hospice and Palliative Medicine, 4700 W Lake Avenue, Glenview, IL 60025; Tel. (847) 375-4712; www. aahpm.org

American Board of Hospice and Palliative Medicine, 9200 Daleview Court, Silver Spring, MD 20901; Tel. (301) 439-8001; www.abhpm.org

American Cancer Society; Tel. (800) 227-2345; www.cancer.org

American Heart Association National Center, 7272 Greenville Avenue, Dallas, TX 75231; Tel. (800-242-8721; www.americanheart.org

American Hospice Foundation, 2120 L Street, NW, Suite 200, Washington, DC 20037; Tel. (202)-223-0204; www.americanhospice.org

American Lung Association, 61 Broadway, 6th Floor, New York, NY 10006; Tel. (800) LUNG-USA; www.lungusa.org

American Medical Association, 515 N. State Street, Chicago, IL 60610; Tel. (800) 621-8335; www.ama-assn.org

American Medical Directors Association, 10480 Little Patuxent Parkway, Suite 760, Columbia, MD 21044; Tel. (410) 740-9743 / (800) 876-2632; www.amda.com

American Nurses Association, 8515 Georgia Avenue, Suite 400, Silver Spring, MD 20910-3492; Tel. (301) 628-5000; www.nursingworld.org

Centers for Disease Control and Prevention, 1600 Clifton Road, Atlanta, GA 30333; Tel: (404) 639-3311 / Public Inquiries: (404) 639-3534 / (800) 311-3435; www.cdc.gov

Centers for Medicare & Medicaid Services, 7500 Security Boulevard, Baltimore, MD 21244-1850; Tel. (877) 267-2323; www.cms.hhs.gov

Detroit Area Agency on Aging, 1333 Brewery Park Boulevard, Suite 200, Detroit, MI 48207; Tel. (313) 446-4444; www.daaa1a.org/DAAA/

Hospice Association of America, 228 Seventh Street, SE, Washington, DC 20003; Tel. (202) 546-4759; www.nahc.org/HAA

Hospice Education Institute, 3 Unity Square, P.O. Box 98, Machiasport, ME 04655-0098; Tel. Hospicelink (800) 331-1620, (207) 255-8800; www.dhospiceworld.org

Hospice and Palliative Nurses Association, Penn Center West One, Suite 229, Pittsburgh, PA 15276; Tel. (412) 787-9301; www.hpna.org

Hospice Foundation of America, 1621 Connecticut Avenue, NW Suite 300, Washington, DC 20009; Tel. (800) 854-3402; www.hospicefoundation.org

Institute of Gerontology, Wayne State University, 87 East Ferry Street, 226 Knapp Building, Detroit, MI 48202, Tel. (313) 577-2297; www.iog.wayne.edu

National Alliance for Caregiving, 4720 Montgomery Lane, 5th Floor, Bethesda, MD 20814; www.caregiving.org

National Association of Health Care Assistants, 1201 L Street NW, Washington, DC 20005; Tel. (202) 454-1288, (800) 784-6049; www.nahcacares.org

National Association of People With AIDS, 8401 Colesville Road, Suite 750, Silver Spring, MD 20910; Tel. (240)-247-0880; www.napwa.org

National Cancer Institute, NCI Public Inquiries Office, 6116 Executive Boulevard, Room 3036A, Bethesda, MD 20892; Tel. (800)-4-CANCER, (800)-422-6237; www.cancer.gov

National Caucus and Center on Black Aged, 1220 L Street NW, Suite 800, Washington DC 20005; Tel. (202) 637-8400; www.ncba-aged.org

National Senior Citizens Law Center, 1101 14th Street NW, Suite 400, Washington DC 20005: Tel. (202) 289-6976 x201; www.nsclc.org

National Citizens' Coalition for Nursing Home Reform, 1828 L Street, NW, Suite 801, Washington, DC 20036; Tel. (202) 332-2276; www.nccnhr.org

National Council on the Aging, 300 D Street, SW, Suite 801, Washington, DC 20024; Tel. (202) 479-1200; www.ncoa.org

National Hospice and Palliative Care Organization (NHPCO), 1700 Diagonal Road, Suite 625, Alexandria, VA 22314; Tel. (800) 658-8898; www.nhpco.org

National Institute of Nursing Research, Bethesda, MD 20892-217; http://ninr.nih.gov/ninr/

National Service-Learning Partnership at the Academy for Educational Development, 1825 Connecticut Avenue, NW-Suite 800, Washington, DC 200095721; Tel. (202) 884-8595; www.service-learningpartnership.org.

National Youth Leadership Council (NYLC), 1667 Snelling Avenue North, Suite D 300, Saint Paul, MN 55108: Tel. (651) 631-3672; www.nylc.org

Social Security Administration, Office of Public Inquiries, Windsor Park Building, 6401 Security Blvd., Baltimore, MD 21235; Tel. (800) 772-1213; www.ssa.gov

The Hastings Center, 21 Malcolm Gordon Road, Garrison, NY 10524-5555; Tel. (845) 424-4040; www.thehastingscenter.org

U.S. Department of Health and Human Services, 200 Independence Avenue, S.W., Washington, DC 20201; Tel. (202) 619-0257, Toll Free: 1-877-696-6775: www.os.dhhs.gov

U.S. Department of Veterans Affairs, Office of Public Affairs (80D), 810 Vermont Avenue, N.W., Washington, DC 20420, Headstones and Markers Tel. (800) 827-1000; www.va.gov

Index

CPSIA information can be obtained at www.ICGtesting.com
Printed in the USA
BVOW08s1655050215

386300BV00004B/65/P

9 781932 690354